KNOWING WHY WE EAT: UNDERSTANDING THE FACTORS INFLUENCING FOOD CHOICES

DISCOVER THE SECRET TO ACHIEVING THE BODY YOU WANT WITH A SIMPLE 7-STEP PLAN

JAIRO HERNANDEZ

CONTENTS

INTRODUCTION

What does "eating healthy" really mean? The obvious answer is a balanced diet that limits processed foods. A diet that is filled with nutritious foods. Yet, if the answer is so obvious, why are so many of us struggling with diet-related health concerns? Surely, we must be missing the bigger picture somehow. Refocusing on the bigger picture is something that I do best, so join me as we go on a journey of discovery.

I am the author of the book, *Knowing What You Think About is Where You Will Go: Making Every Day Count*, and a retired military veteran who served over two decades with honorable military service. In my previous written work, I realized that many people limit their true potential and block themselves through self-sabotage. "It has to do with what we think about and how we choose to put our dreams into motion; you can have the most fantastic plan in place, and it can still fall apart." Not surprisingly, many people approach the concept of healthy eating with the same level of self-sabotage. Although, when it comes to food, that sabotage may not always be intentional or obvious.

Knowing Why We Eat: Understanding the Factors Influencing Food Choices is an abridgment of my previous works, in which the goal or objective will fall into place when we understand why we think the way we think. We will have a better chance of achieving the desired health goal if we know which foods work for us. It could be for disease prevention, weight management, or simply to live a longer, healthier life.

While serving in the military, I was physically active. Eating healthy was ingrained into my mind and body within a high-tempo military lifestyle. This is how I was able to survive daily military life. During my time as a military service member, I tried to understand why we eat the way we do and what foods are the best for my body composition. Foods that help our minds and bodies function optimally. I looked at all the different diet types, from high protein intake to intermittent fasting, to juicing, to adding supplemental nutrition to my diet. You name it, and I tried it. My goal was to keep my body at optimal performance for long runs and trekking in unpredictable terrain. There are many physical demands of military life and combat outside the country, and keeping my body in optimal condition was a priority.

Embracing a New Approach to Life

As a result of all my experimentation, I grew to understand the importance of having a healthy diet for your mind and body to perform at their best. Due to my Mexican culture, I had to change what foods worked best for me because of my high cholesterol. The discovery of my high cholesterol came as a shock, as I was the picture of health: trim and fit! As a result, I experimented with foods and finally found what worked for my body. In this process, I uncovered a simple but powerful truth: You must eat balanced meals that include all the nutrients your body needs for your body composition and biochemistry.

Achieving a healthy weight is the missing piece of the puzzle, and it requires understanding your relationship with food. This relationship is formed in our childhood through culture and psychology. I believe anyone can have the body they deserve to live a healthier life without needing to be on a strict diet plan. That's right! You don't need to follow an oppressive fad diet when you understand your relationship with food. Instead, you'll learn to enjoy the foods that give the body the best nutrients for optimal performance.

What You Will Learn

In this book, you'll discover the real meaning of "eating healthy." Here's a quick spoiler alert: Fad diets and meal plans are not as helpful as we might assume. We don't need to disregard meal plans entirely though. You can use diet plans on the market to help you lay the experimental foundations you can use to then figure out what works for you and your whole family. This book will help reacquaint us with the basics of nutrition, while encouraging us to take a deeper look at our relationship with food.

When it comes to improving your health and well-being, scientifically changing your mindset about food will make a difference. Eating the right foods for your body composition will prevent diseases from forming and enable you to live your best life without putting too much pressure on yourself. You deserve to look and feel your best while loving the skin you're in!

We will go through the cultural and psychological reasons that drive our food choices. Furthermore, you'll learn how to tap into the biochemistry of nutrition and how it may, or may not, work for your body chemistry.

With six simple questions you'll be able to reclaim control over your eating habits and food choices and kickstart your 7-step plan. This journey into the world of food education will turn everything you think you know about nutrition on its head. The only question that now remains is this: Are you ready to discover a world of possibility?

F4URY.COM was founded by me. The focus of F4URY is on empowering people from all walks of life to live healthy, wealthy, and happy lives. Everyone can strive for greatness; it is much more attainable than you think!

1

THE SEVEN FACTORS THAT INFLUENCE YOUR FOOD CHOICES

We all want to make healthy choices. But how? We often make poor choices because we don't know how to make healthy ones. Sometimes we are unaware of all the things that influence our choices. Many factors influence our food choices. These factors include our family history, genetics, environment, culture, and social circle. Many people eat unhealthy foods because their environments are filled with fast food, soda, and junk food. Perhaps their parents and grandparents were raised on junk food when they were young. Now, they are still teaching this to their children and grandchildren. Many cultural norms and traditional eating habits also influence eating.

Basic economic theories state that most people purchase food and other marketplace goods to maximize utility. It makes sense. We want to get the most value for our money, especially in difficult economic times. Under the constraint that the price is below or equal to the amount of all the sources of income, what we buy depends on our preferences. Income limitations and time restrictions for preparing food have made it difficult for households to buy healthy food.

Events and experiences have a strong influence on our food choices. These influences start early in life and continue throughout it. Understanding how food choices occur justifies a deeper investigation. We need to look at these choices from the perspective of the life course. A life course refers to an individual's past experiences related to multiple trajectories, transitions, and turning points and the context in which they occurred. Food choices are influenced by both the life course and current influences. Simply put, the way we eat is influenced by many factors that we don't usually consider.

An overview of cultural beliefs about eating healthy and how they were developed is needed. Food is a necessary part of retaining culture. For example, we won't associate sushi with Mexico. So, food speaks volumes about where we come from and, in essence, who we are. Certain cultures are believed to be healthier than others, and some people believe some countries have a better diet. The truth is that food is a celebration of culture, and different cultures can enjoy their favorite dishes if they know how to cook better. Like it or not, our food preferences are affected by social norms, learning behaviors, and evolutionary processes.

Where we live and the families we grow up in have a big impact on our food preferences and dislikes. One family's delicacy might be another's kitchen nightmare. Take durian fruit as an example. This melon-sized spiky fruit has a potent smell but is widely consumed by families in Southeast Asia. The scent might be offensive, but the taste seems to be worth it. Then again, many American families are fond of canned spray cheese, a product that certainly raises a few eyebrows in other countries. The debate about cultural food differences is a fascinating one and can fill a library on its own. In this chapter, we'll take a closer look at the social, biological, economic, and physical factors that influence the way we eat.

SOCIAL FACTORS THAT INFLUENCE FOOD CHOICE

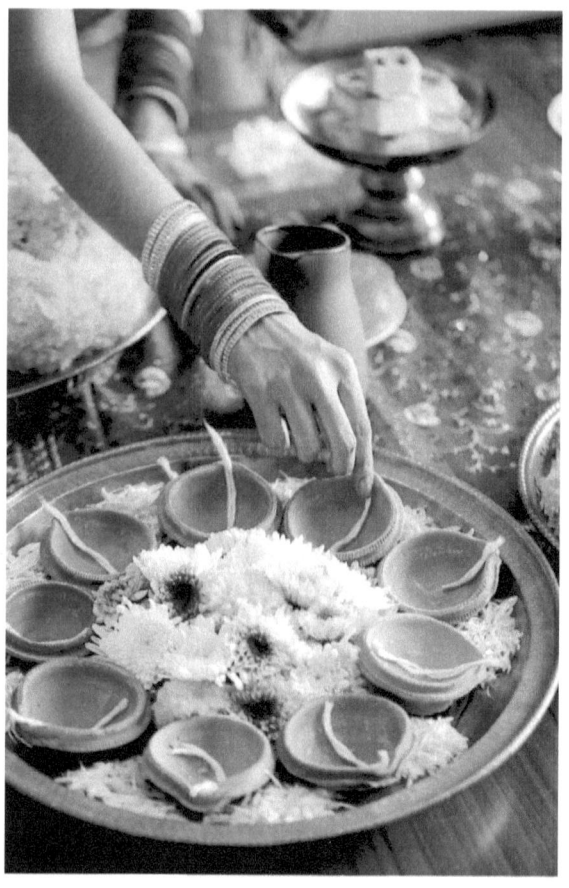

As social beings, food plays a big part in our lives. A person's cultural and social background can affect their food choices. The traditional foods of their culture, the foods they were exposed to growing up, and the foods they eat with friends and family can all be included.

Understanding how the people we dine with influence what we eat becomes all the more important. A lot of what we eat takes place in a social context. From decades of research, we know that other people influence our food choices and intake. When we eat with someone who consumes a lot of food, we are more likely to mimic their eating pattern and eat more than we usually would (Ruddock et al., 2019). That being said, let's take a closer look at the different social factors that influence our eating behaviors.

Cultural Influence on Food Choice

Social context strongly influences how we eat. We eat differently around people we know and don't know. Social acceptance and competing norms are important factors in this. For example, if a romantic partner hates tomatoes on their burger, we are more likely to order ours without them as well. Even though we like tomatoes on our burgers, we are modeling our eating after the person we look up to. This is norm matching, but there are limitations to this. Let's say that the same partner wants something unusual on his burger (for example, durian fruit), we'd likely order our burger the way we usually do.

Norm matching is a subtle process that involves synchronization of eating action, watching what we eat, and altering food preferences. Next time you eat with a friend, loved one, or co-worker, take note of the subtle ways in which your eating behavior differs from when you are eating alone. Chances are, if the person or group is eating a lot, you'll eat more than you normally would too. On the flip side, if the group we are dining with sticks to small portions, we are more likely to adopt a matched eating behavior. This is called modeling, and it is a well-studied phenomenon. Modeling can present itself in different ways, but it is important to understand that it is a norm that is set by another.

Understanding Modeling

Children and adults tend to model the eating behaviors of others, but there are exceptions to the rule. Studies found that women who score high in impulsivity do not easily copy other people's eating behaviors (Hermans et al., 2012). The study suggests that our degree of impulsivity could influence how we eat. Yet another study found that individuals who score low in the self-control department are far more likely to model their eating behaviors after those of their peers (Salmon et al., 2014).

These findings seem contradictory, but keep in mind that the research methods in these studies differed, making it difficult to compare. Most likely, unmeasured variables had a hand in the results of both studies. However, the findings help us unravel the complex reasons why we eat the way we do. Human behavior is complex, so it would be unreasonable to expect a single study to cover all bases. One thing is certain, though: When we are concerned with behaving in a socially appropriate way, we are far more likely to copy the eating behaviors of others (Cavazza et al., 2011). Just think of all the times you, a friend, or an acquaintance adjusted eating behavior in unfamiliar surroundings.

Not only do models affect our eating behaviors—for example, by altering our food choices to match those of the people around us—but they also dictate how much we eat at times. When our companions eat small portions, we are likely to follow suit because we feel it is appropriate in that situation. Try to recall all the situations where you ate less than you normally would. It could have been on a date, at a work function, at a social event, or even at a friend's house. You probably thought that eating less was the right thing to do at the time. That's because we are more likely to adjust the amount of food we eat around people we identify with (Stok et al., 2013). This also means that if the person we look up to has a big appetite, we'll likely eat more too.

The Role of Preferences

Copying our peers's eating behaviors is not the only thing that changes the way we eat. Ninety percent of our serotonin receptors are located in the gut (Sawhney, 2021). As an important neurotransmitter, serotonin plays a key role in sleep, digestion, bone health, and mood regulation. When our serotonin levels are too high or too low, it can trigger a range of physical and psychological problems (*Serotonin*, 2022). Food can impact our mood in a big way by encouraging or hindering gut health. The food we consume has a direct impact on gut health and, by extension, the production of neurotransmitters.

Serotonin also influences our mood, which explains why we reach for comfort food on certain occasions. Comfort food makes us feel good because it triggers the release of serotonin and dopamine. So, foods have the power to trigger emotions and physiological changes (Sawhney, 2021). For example, our taste buds contain VR1 receptors. These receptors detect heat and lead to sweating and discomfort when activated (Sawhney, 2021).

Food's impact on the body (emotionally and physically) becomes even more important in a social context. Studies found that conforming to a group norm can be a rewarding experience (Klucharev et al., 2009). Shared experiences are amplified, so eating with someone becomes more pleasurable (Boothby et al., 2014).

The Power of Environmental Cues

Can your surroundings change your eating habits? Environmental cues can be subtle but powerful. Take those free chocolates in coffee shops or work lunch rooms as an example. How often do we help ourselves to them? According to researchers, if there's evidence of consumption (empty wrappers) in the environment, we'd likely reach for the chocolates too (Prinsen et al., 2013).

Empty wrappers near free chocolates aren't the only environmental cues that can tempt us to eat. The holidays, celebrations, events, and family gatherings can influence what we eat in positive or negative ways. There are many occasions when our food choices are influenced, for example:

- Enjoying hot dogs with a barbeque.
- Eating lunch at your workstation or computer.
- Indulging in ice cream on a hot day.
- Having s'mores when camping.
- Indulging in cookies, candies and treats on holidays.

Being aware of these influences and identifying them is an important step in making healthy food choices. Useful strategies can help us replace unhelpful food cues with healthy choices (Earnesty, 2018). For example, if we have a habit of eating at the computer, a simple sticky note on the screen can remind us to eat our lunch or dinner elsewhere. Keeping fresh fruit and vegetables at eye level in the refrigerator can help us make healthier choices too. Recognizing food cues in our environment can help us adopt healthy behaviors and maintain a healthy weight.

The Link Between Social Norms and Obesity

People who are socially connected (friends and family) tend to make similar eating choices (Barclay et al., 2013). This means that if we have friends or family whose normal food choice is to overeat (or eat unhealthy food), we'd likely follow suit. This adoption of other people's eating habits can explain why clusters of obesity can be found in social circles (Stockman, 2009). Of course, we can't discount changes in our levels of physical activity or perceptions about body sizes, as these all play a role in the formation of social norms.

Social norms can play a significant role in the rise of obesity. It does so by enforcing new eating patterns. For example, the average portion size in American restaurants has tripled over the last two decades (*Larger Portion Sizes Contribute to U.S. Obesity Problem*, 2013). Super-sized portions have certainly contributed to distorting our perception of what a "normal" portion size should be. In many cases, these large meals can add up to 1,500 additional calories per day to our diet, leading to weight gain. This increase in average portion size does not remain in the restaurant we dine at; it is a value that bleeds through our social networks as well (Peter Herman et al., 2015). Part of the reason for this can be attributed to the fact that the social context of eating changed. People are far more likely to overeat now than in the past. With more people eating at fast food outlets, we may be more susceptible to environmental cues than before (Vartanian et al., 2013).

Social Class Influence on Food Choice

The influence of social class on food choices is an important topic. Social class is how individuals are grouped based on their economic status. A person's education level and income are referred to as their "social class." It is more likely that the person will have better health and a better diet if they are in a high social class. The cost of healthy food is one of the reasons for poor eating patterns among low-income households. A growing body of evidence shows that the purchase and consumption of unhealthy foods are strongly linked to socio-economic status (Appelhans et al., 2012).

The cost of food is the likely driving force behind most food purchases, with energy-dense foods being cheaper and high-quality foods (like whole grains, whole foods, raw foods, and preservative-free foods) being more costly. As a result, the food we eat reflects our preferences and socio-economic status.

Imagine this scenario: You have $10.00 and want to buy a muffin. Let's say a whole-grain or gluten-free muffin costs $5.00, whereas a regular chocolate chip muffin is priced at $1.40. Which muffin would you go for? It's likely we'd go for the cheaper muffin, simply because we can fit more of them (roughly seven) into our budget. Now let's take that same scenario, but this time we have $100.00 to spend. We'd probably choose the whole-grain or gluten-free muffin this time around because we can afford it. So, dietary costs explain a big part of the relationship between socio-economic status and the food we consume (Monsivais et al., 2010). That is only part of the picture, though, as the relationship between socio-economic status and the food we eat seems to be a bi-directional one.

Our socio-economic status impacts which kinds of foods we can afford, but at the same time, our education and preferences play a part too. Studies found that consumers who frequent low-priced supermarkets will more likely have a lower-quality diet, but educated households are able to make healthier purchases within the same store (Handbury et al., 2015). In other words, even though our food choices are limited in low-priced supermarkets, we'd still be able to make healthier food choices if we were aware of our options. Also, preferences play an important role. Sometimes we may choose to buy from retailers that offer superior products or services. This choice is not free from monetary implications, though. Our socio-economic status influences the types of goods we can afford (Pechey et al., 2015). Simply put, socio-economic status and awareness of available options are a big reason why food poverty exists.

Peers's Influence on Food Choice

Does the following situation sound familiar? You are grabbing a bite to eat with friends at a local bar. Everyone in the group orders either a pizza, a half-pound burger, or a quarter chicken with fries. You are eyeing the menu, and the salad looks nice. For a brief moment, you consider ordering it, but you realize your friends will mock you for being on a "diet." You decide to order a burger instead. Before you know it, you are uncomfortably full and reaching for antacids. Evidence suggests that this behavior is not unusual. When we dine with others, we tend to follow the crowd (Zimmerle, 2022).

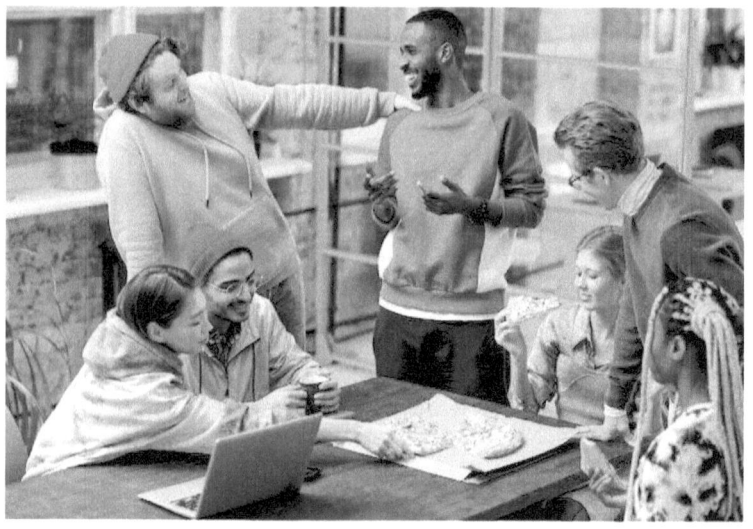

Researchers investigating the impact of peer pressure on our eating habits found that we adjust our eating habits to fit in with the group. Sometimes we don't realize the impact that our friends can have on our eating habits, and we may end up copying them even when we are eating alone. But peer pressure does not have to be a bad thing! As one study points out, the desire to fit in can be harnessed for good. The study found that people who saw their coworkers eat their fruits and vegetables were more likely to eat them too (van der Put & Ellwardt, 2022).

Not surprisingly, the social impact that food carries is not limited to physical spaces. Social media can have an impact on our eating habits. In a 2020 study, researchers found that social media users who observe their peers' eating habits online are more likely to eat extra portions of fruit, vegetables, or junk food (Hawkins et al., 2020). Sounds strange? Try to recall all the times you felt like nibbling on something after you saw posts from your foodie friends online. Chances are you've helped yourself to something tasty (or wanted to) after seeing a few of those scrumptious-looking posts!

Health Consequences

If your friends and family eat unhealthy food, you're more likely to eat unhealthy food as well. Peer pressure influences people to make unhealthy food choices, which is a direct impact, while learning from the behavior of others has an indirect effect. All of this has the potential to impact our waistlines significantly. A 2007 study found that individuals who have a close friend who is obese are at an increased risk of becoming obese themselves (Kolata, 2007). Similar findings have been reported when siblings or spouses are obese. We unconsciously eat differently when surrounded by other people than when we eat alone. Our dietary choices tend to merge with those we are close to in our social connections. Social support (e.g., family) can help you cope with the negative feelings you experience when you are alone by encouraging healthy eating habits.

BIOLOGICAL INFLUENCE ON FOOD CHOICE

There is a vast difference between how we think about food and how it makes us feel. Many of us don't realize how what we eat affects our brain and hormones. This in turn affects our moods and overall well-being. Some foods can be used as medicine, such as making ginger tea to relieve digestive problems. Other foods, such as junk food, are not as helpful and can be harmful.

The factors that influence food choices are hunger, appetite, and satiety. Everyone's characteristics are unique and can change a lot. Your flavor experience is constructed into your genes. These begin to develop during the first six months of a baby's life and play a role in the development of food choices later in life. We tend to like sweet things and don't like bitter or sour things.

The structure and function of the brain influence our food choices as well. Specifically, the hypothalamus and the reward system. The hypothalamus plays a big part in appetite regulation, so taking care of it is very important. The reward system, which is triggered by pleasurable stimulation, can also influence what we eat. Certain foods can cause the release of pleasure-inducing chemicals like dopamine. This is part of the reason why we enjoy sweet treats. Sugar triggers the release of dopamine, which can make us crave more of it (Reichelt, 2019). In this section, we'll take a closer look at the biology that drives our food choices.

Hunger Signals

These signals are physiological cues that tell the brain you need to eat. Hunger signals originate from the hypothalamus, a small brain region responsible for regulating hunger and satiety. While the hypothalamus is a small structure located deep in the brain, it is an important one. Heart rate, body temperature, and hunger are all controlled by the hypothalamus. The body uses several hunger signals to stimulate appetite. These signals are:

- **Ghrelin:** Ghrelin, or the "hunger hormone" is produced by the stomach and increases hunger by stimulating the hypothalamus.

- **Low blood sugar:** When the body's blood sugar levels drop, the hypothalamus sends signals to the brain to eat to raise blood sugar levels.
- **Stomach contractions:** When the stomach is empty, it signals to the hypothalamus that the body needs food.
- **The smell and sight of food:** The nose's olfactory receptors and the eyes' visual receptors can detect the scent and sight of food, stimulating appetite.
- **Hormonal changes:** Hormones such as cortisol and insulin can also influence hunger signals. High levels of cortisol and low levels of insulin can stimulate hunger.

It is possible to miss hunger cues entirely. Whenever we eat out of boredom, while watching Netflix, or based on social cues, we are not really paying attention to physical hunger signals. Reclaiming our eating habits starts by recognizing physical hunger cues and the cues for satiation. Mindfulness is key.

Mindfulness is defined as focusing your attention on the present moment. In a state of mindfulness, the past and future do not exist; you only have the here and now. Mindfulness is about paying attention to your immediate surroundings without passing judgment. It is not meditation. Paying close attention to what you eat through mindfulness can help us recognize hunger and satiety cues and help build an appreciation for the food we eat (Pope, 2021). Ask yourself these simple questions the next time you grab a bite to eat to evaluate how hungry you really are:

- Do I feel hungry or thirsty?
- If I'm feeling hungry, how hungry am I on a scale from 1–10? (10 being not hungry at all).
- Do I want to eat this food item? If not, what do I want to eat?
- Is this food item nutritious?
- How do I feel (physically and emotionally)?

Determining when you are full (but not uncomfortably stuffed) can be hard, but the tips below can help us reconnect with our bodies.

- **Exercise regularly to encourage a healthy metabolism.** A healthy metabolism makes it much easier for us to recognize hunger and satiation cues. Keep in mind that the average individual needs roughly 150 minutes of exercise per week, but it is advised to speak to your healthcare provider if you have any concerns.

- **Stay hydrated.** Drinking enough water can help prevent overeating. Many times, we mistake our thirst for hunger, which leads to extra (and unneeded) calories being added to our bodies. The average healthy adult living in a temperate climate needs about 8 cups of water daily (*Water: How Much Should You Drink Every Day?*, 2020). Usually, you can tell if you are drinking enough water when you don't feel thirsty or if your urine is colorless or light yellow.

- **Eat off of smaller plates.** Smaller plates teach us portion control, but there's another reason to embrace smaller dinnerware. Some people have a tendency to eat everything on their plate. This is not necessarily a bad thing, but polishing off a large amount of food simply because it is on your plate is not doing your body any favors. By using smaller plates and bowls, these individuals can still finish their food without overeating.

- **Chewing your food slowly will help you feel fuller quicker.** That's because when we take our time to chew food properly, our bodies can produce leptin. Leptin is produced in the fat cells and signals the brain that we are full. When we unceremoniously scarf down our food, we don't give our bodies time to register the amount of food we've eaten, which often leads to overeating.

Appetite Senses

Appetite senses refer to the body's physiological mechanisms to sense hunger and satiety, the desire to eat, and the feeling of fullness. These mechanisms help regulate food intake and energy balance in the body. Several appetite senses are involved in the regulation of food intake:

- **Sight:**

The sight of food can stimulate appetite, as the brain associates specific visual cues with the taste and smell of food. Some researchers believe that humans evolved color vision to help them find energy-rich foods. Today, we simply walk into a grocery store to find our food, but we still use our eyes. Just think of all the times you avoided a tomato or banana that looked overripe! We constantly forage with our eyes in supermarkets to find the best-looking produce.

- **Smell:**

The smell of food can also stimulate appetite, as the olfactory receptors in the nose can detect the volatile compounds in food and send signals to the brain. Most scientists believe that a good portion of our taste is derived from our sense of smell. This is part of the reason why food tastes so darn bland when we have a cold or flu. But aromas do more than alert us to a tasty dish in the vicinity. Scent has the power to sway our food choices. For example, people who smelled melon or pear without knowing it were more likely to order vegetable dishes or fruit-based desserts with their meal (Mikstas, 2021). In the food industry, this tidbit is worth its weight in gold, as the right scents have the potential to increase food sales by 300% (Yu, 2017). This results in a lot of unintentional calories being consumed.

- **Taste:**

The taste of food is detected by the taste buds on the tongue, which can detect sweet, sour, salty, and bitter flavors. These taste receptors send signals to the brain, influencing food choices and appetite. The way food looks can influence our taste experience in interesting ways. Studies indicate that we perceive food as tastier when it is plated attractively (Zellner et al., 2014). Plating foods attractively is one way we can make healthy foods more palatable.

- **Touch:**

The texture of food can also influence appetite, as the sensation of crunching or softness can affect how appealing a portion of food is perceived to be. Texture can influence taste in a number of ways. For example, the thickness of a food item can influence how strong it tastes. We also equate crispy food items (like potato chips) with saltiness and fattiness, which many people have been conditioned to want (Heavner, 2019). Sour candies are often coated in rough sugar to enhance the taste (people tend to perceive rough foods as being more sour). Texture plays a big role in what we eat and how much we eat, and manufacturers of processed and junk foods know this. It is through a combination of salt, fat, and crispness that chip manufacturers get us to devour entire bags in one sitting. It is a combination that is very hard to resist, but the power of texture can be used to make healthy foods more appealing too.

Our senses affect what we eat in the most amazing ways. Something as simple as the weight of the dish can influence our taste experience. Researchers found that when people are given a food item (like yogurt) in a heavier bowl, they consistently rate that item as more appealing and higher in quality (Piqueras-Fiszman et al., 2011). Next time you are enjoying some yogurt, serve it in a heavy bowl. You might be pleasantly surprised at the difference this simple adjustment can make!

Palatability of Taste

The enjoyment or appeal of food and drink is referred to as the palatability of taste. It is a subjective measure of how appealing or desirable a food or drink is based on its taste, smell, texture, and appearance. Personal preferences, cultural backgrounds, experiences, and learned behaviors can also be influenced by palatability.

Palatability plays a key role in food choice and food intake, as people are more likely to eat foods that are considered palatable. However, palatability alone does not determine food choice. The nutritional value, availability, cost, and other factors also influence it. Understanding what influences palatability is a useful step when developing strategies to encourage healthy food choices. Not surprisingly, genetics influences palatability.

Findings from recent research found that taste-related genes can influence our food choices. This study is among the first to examine how genetics and taste (sweet, salty, bitter, sour, and umami) are linked to our food consumption. One interesting finding that surfaced in the study is that people who have a strong taste perception of bitter flavors tend to eat less cruciferous vegetables like cauliflower, kale, bok choy, and cabbage (Henderson, 2022). These foods typically contain a beneficial compound called glucosinolates. This compound is responsible for the bitter taste and the many health benefits linked to these vegetables. However, people who strongly perceive bitter tastes may find these foods less palatable. Findings suggest that individuals who strongly perceive bitter and umami tastes tend to eat fewer whole grains and vegetables. It should be noted that while genetics play an important role in how we perceive taste, the findings of this study can't be generalized to everyone, and a deeper investigation is needed into the link between genetics and food preferences.

ECONOMIC INFLUENCE ON FOOD CHOICE

Income levels don't seem to affect nutrition knowledge, but you have more access to healthier and more diverse foods as you become more prosperous. This trend is becoming more visible as the global food price crisis continues. The World Health Organization notes that the global food price crises threaten public health and impact women, children, the elderly, and low-income families the most (Yt et al., 2009). With the global poverty line placed at $2.15 per person, per day, it becomes easy to see how economic factors influence food choices (*Fact Sheet: An Adjustment to Global Poverty Lines*, n.d.).

Rising food prices have a severe impact on our health and well-being. This is why we see a range of nutrition-ally-related disorders and diseases cropping up in individuals who changed their diet for economic reasons. This happens more frequently than we'd like to think about, with one in every four individuals suffering from moderate to severe food insecurity globally (Roser & Ritchie, 2013). The inability to purchase affordable, healthy foods is one of the biggest problems tied to income-related food insecurity. Low-income families can't afford to make healthy food choices because of the cost. Even if they can afford more nutritious options, they may buy fewer healthy options because they are more affordable. Financial assistance to purchase food can help alleviate some of the economic barriers.

On the flip side, if you have a healthy bank balance but don't know anything about healthy eating and nutrition, that won't help you either! Yes, you'll be able to afford healthy food items, but the lack of food education may lead you to make unhealthy choices. A study investigating the link between income and fast-food purchases found that rich people like to indulge in fast food as well. Nearly three-quarters (75%) of wealthy participants in the study admitted to visiting fast-food establishments (Fearnow, 2017).

A combination of education and affordable healthy foods is, therefore, needed to address the worrying trend of unhealthy food consumption and the health problems it brings. Below, we'll take a brief look at three of the biggest economic factors that influence our food choices.

- **Expense of food:**

The average cost for a healthy diet per person per day is estimated to be $3.54 (*Food Prices for Nutrition DataHub: Global Statistics on the Cost and Affordability of Healthy Diets*, n.d.). With the global poverty line pegged at $2.15 per person per day, one doesn't need to be a mathematician to realize that eating healthy is simply unaffordable for many people. In fact, more than three billion people worldwide can't afford the average cost of a healthy diet (*The State of Food Security and Nutrition in the World 2022*, 2022). The cost of food can make it challenging to eat healthy, regardless of how healthy your bank balance is. Fortunately, there are ways we can introduce healthy foods into our diet without breaking the bank. Growing our own produce whenever possible, buying in bulk, planning meals, cooking at home, shopping from local markets, and bargain hunting online are all viable strategies to get more value for a thinly stretched income.

- **Income variability:**

Food insecurity can be either long- or short-term and may be related to income factors and employment. We want to eat healthy for many reasons. These reasons can include improving our health, saving money, looking good, and being happier. Those with higher incomes can afford more quality and diverse foods, while those with lower incomes have fewer choices. In 2020, more than a quarter (28.6%) of low-income American households were classified as food insecure (*Food Insecurity*, n.d.). Racial and ethnic differences also seem to contribute to the risk of food insecurity with African American and Hispanic households having an increased risk. Other factors that influence food security include the neighborhood we live in, transportation (or the lack thereof), and accessibility of food. We'll discuss food accessibility in the next point.

- **Accessibility and availability of food:**

Food deserts come to mind when discussing the accessibility and availability of food. Food deserts refer to areas, typically urban, where it is difficult to access affordable and fresh food. These food deserts can originate because there aren't a lot of shopping facilities around or because the food available is too expensive. Improving access and eradicating food deserts does not mean people will change their habits, though. Although many of us can order our food online, or grow bunches of spinach in the garden, the lack of access to healthy food remains a significant barrier to public health. When we don't eat vegetables of all types, grains (preferably whole grain), fruits, dairy, protein, and healthy fats, we put ourselves at risk for developing diet-related chronic diseases (*Access to Foods That Support Healthy Dietary Patterns*, n.d.). When you live in a food desert, it may be difficult to access a grocery store that sells healthy foods. Fortunately, it's easier than ever to improve the availability of fresh fruits and vegetables in low-income and rural areas. Online shopping, food education, and basic gardening knowledge can go a long way toward improving the conditions we find in food deserts.

PHYSICAL FACTORS INFLUENCE ON FOOD CHOICE

Personal factors such as age, gender, taste preferences, and dietary restrictions also play a role in food choices. Everyone's characteristics are unique and can vary greatly. A person's level of education strongly influences adult dietary behavior. Unlike nutrition knowledge and good dietary habits, which are not strongly correlated. This is because information about health does not compel individuals to take direct action when they are unsure how to apply it. Furthermore, nutrition information comes from various sources that can be ambiguous and inconsistent. This discourages motivation to change, so accurate and consistent messages about nutrition must be conveyed through multiple media—on food packages and by health professionals.

Many people make food choices based on convenience rather than nutrition. Take New York as an example. Thousands of New Yorkers live in food deserts and are reliant on their local corner store to buy food, as larger grocery stores are too far away or too expensive (Walsh, 2022). These corner stores typically sell convenient microwaveable meals and junk foods. So, the food options available in an area, the ease of preparation, and the time it takes to prepare a meal are all factors that influence food choices. An important factor that needs to be examined closer is our knowledge about food nutrition.

Education and Knowledge

Knowledge about food and nutrition influences how you make food choices. People who know more about nutrition tend to make healthier food choices and are more likely to understand the importance of eating various nutritious foods. Hence, they get all the essential nutrients they need for good health. Understanding nutrition refers to an individual's knowledge of the relationship between food and health. Those with more knowledge about food and nutrition tend to eat healthier foods and are more likely to understand the importance of a balanced diet. People who are more aware of the dangers of eating certain foods or engaging in certain food practices are more conscious of what they eat.

- **Understanding nutrient needs:** Knowing the types and amounts of nutrients the body needs for optimal health can help individuals make informed food choices.
- **Knowledge of food groups:** Understanding the different food groups, such as fruits and vegetables, grains, proteins, and dairy, and their

role in a healthy diet can help individuals make balanced food choices.

- **Knowledge of food labeling:** Understanding how to read and interpret food labels can help individuals make informed choices about the foods they consume.

- **Knowledge of food safety:** Understanding how to properly store, prepare, and handle food to prevent food-borne illness can help individuals make healthy food choices.

- **Understanding portion sizes:** Understanding appropriate portion sizes can help individuals make informed choices about the amount of food they consume.

- **Knowledge of cooking and meal preparation:** Understanding how to cook and prepare healthy meals can help individuals make healthier food choices.

- **Knowledge of food-related diseases:** Understanding the link between diet and disease and how certain foods can impact health can help individuals make healthier food choices.

- **Knowledge of food budgeting:** Understanding how to budget for healthy food options can help individuals make healthier food choices.

Education and knowledge about healthy eating can empower individuals to make informed choices about their diet and promote overall health (Kana"An et al., 2021). As a bonus, food education can also help us save money in the long run.

ATTITUDES, BELIEFS, AND BEHAVIORS ABOUT FOOD SELECTION

Culture, personal experience, and nutrition knowledge are some of the factors that can affect people's attitudes toward food. Some people value the pleasure of eating and view food as an essential part of social gatherings. After all, the holidays are not the same without delicious food! Others might view food as a necessary fuel to sustain life and place a greater emphasis on weight loss. It's important to remember that people's attitudes about nutrition may not align with what is considered healthy. We are all subject to biases or misconceptions that can affect our food choices. This is why it is essential to educate yourself on actual nutrition facts. A healthcare professional or registered dietitian can be a great source of information. They can help determine if people's attitudes prevent them from making healthier food choices.

All About the Attitudes

Attitudes refer to an individual's feelings and opinions about food and its role. Moods can be positive or negative and vary significantly from person to person. For example, some people may view food as a source of pleasure and enjoyment, while others may view it as a necessary fuel to sustain life. Personal experiences and cultural background can also influence attitudes. Attitudes toward food refer to the individual's beliefs and values about food and its role, as shown in the examples below.

- Positive attitudes towards organic and nonGMO foods, as these are believed to be healthier and more environmentally friendly.
- Negative attitudes about fast food are often seen as high in calories and unhealthy.
- A positive attitude may be a balanced diet involving fruits and vegetables, lean meat, and whole grains.
- Have a negative attitude towards consuming animal products based on ethical and environmental concerns.

Unraveling our attitudes toward food is a complex and rewarding task. After all, knowing your relationship with food has the power to change your life. Our relationship with food is constantly developing throughout our lifetimes. Like all good relationships, a healthy relationship with food is something that needs to be nurtured. Understanding what contributes to an unhealthy relationship with food is an important step. Here are some warning signs to watch out for:

- Developing self-imposed rules around foods that you cannot consume, i.e., believing you can't eat full fat yogurt because it is "fattening." Allergies and medical concerns are a different story.
- Relying extensively on calorie counters and apps (like MyFitnessPal, Noom, and others) to determine when you are done eating for the day. There is nothing wrong with watching what you eat, but it is worrisome if you need an app to tell you you've eaten enough for the day.
- Experiencing feelings of guilt when eating.
- Ignoring your body's hunger and satiation cues.
- Having a history of following fad diets or yo-yo dieting.
- Portion control is challenging and presents concerns over having too little or too much food on the plate.

Eating in social settings may trigger stress or anxiety. Fear of what others will think or say about your food choices could fuel this experience (*What is your attitude and relationship with food?*, 2021).

As with all relationships, not all the red flags need to be present for it to be unhealthy. You could be struggling with portion control or simply feel uncomfortable eating in social settings. However, the road to healing starts by becoming aware of our unhealthy behaviors that inform our attitudes. The ultimate goal of a healthy attitude toward food is to have more positive experiences than bad ones. Remember to be kind to yourself and honest with yourself as you reflect on your relationship with food. So many relationships, business deals, and great ideas originated around the dinner table. As humans, our social lives are built on the tasty foundation of food, so it becomes ever more important to start building a healthy relationship with it. The following indicators indicate a healthy food relationship:

- Listening to and respecting your body's hunger and satiation cues. In other words, you eat when you are hungry and stop when you've had enough, regardless if there is still food on the plate.

- There are no "forbidden" foods, except when allergies or health concerns are present.
- All foods are enjoyed in moderation, except when allergies or health concerns are present. For example, people who are lactose intolerant or sensitive to gluten will avoid certain foods (like dairy and wheat) but still enjoy other foods.
- Other people's opinion of your food choices doesn't influence what you choose to eat, nor do you feel the need to explain why you eat what you eat.
- You've developed an understanding that the food you eat does not define you and choose foods that are good for you.
- Your food choices are not driven by calories.

Keep in mind that your attitude toward and relationship with food are not necessarily tied to your personal health beliefs. It is entirely possible for one to be vegan, pescetarian, or vegetarian and still have a healthy relationship with food. What is important is to examine the behaviors and beliefs that inform our attitudes toward food.

Your Beliefs

Beliefs are convictions or acceptances of something as true or real. They can also influence food choices. For example, a person may believe that certain foods are good for their health or that organic foods are always better than conventional foods. These beliefs can shape food choices and food preferences.

- A belief that a diet high in fruits and vegetables can help prevent chronic diseases.
- The belief that eating meat is bad for the environment.
- Might believe that certain foods, such as gluten or lactose, can cause adverse health effects.
- The belief is that consuming a diet based on one's cultural or religious guidelines is essential.

The Behaviors of Eating Healthy

Behaviors of food choice refer to the actions and decisions people make when it comes to selecting and consuming food. Understanding food choice behaviors can help us better understand the influences on our food choices.

- **Meal planning and preparation:** Planning out meals in advance and preparing them at home, using ingredients that align with one's attitudes and beliefs about food selection.
- **Grocery shopping:** Choosing to shop at certain stores or buy certain brands of food based on one's attitudes and beliefs about food selection, such as buying organic produce or avoiding processed foods.
- **Eating out:** Making conscious choices about where to eat and what to order when eating out, based on one's attitudes and beliefs about food selection, such as choosing a restaurant that serves organic or locally-sourced food or avoiding fast food restaurants.
- **Snacking:** Choosing to snack on healthy options such as fruits, vegetables, nuts, or seeds, rather than processed or high-calorie snacks.
- **Portion control:** Pay attention to the amount of food consumed at each meal, trying to eat until you are satisfied but not overfull.
- **They are avoiding certain foods:** Avoiding certain foods due to allergies, sensitivities, or dietary restrictions, such as gluten or lactose.
- **A dietary guideline:** Follow specific nutritional guidelines such as a Mediterranean diet, a low-carb diet, or a high-protein diet.

- **Cooking methods:** Choosing specific cooking methods, such as steaming, grilling, or baking instead of frying or sautéing, to make healthier choices.
- **Food tracking:** Keeping track of the food consumed, the calories, the macronutrients, and the micronutrients to help make better food choices. In other words, using apps like MyFitnessPal, Noom, and others in a healthy way to make informed food choices, not as a gatekeeper of calories.

These are just a few examples of food choice behaviors, and individuals may engage in a combination of these behaviors based on their attitudes and beliefs about food selection.

ADVERTISING AND MARKETING

The food industry spends billions of dollars on advertising and marketing to influence food choices. In 2016, food companies spent roughly $13.5 billion to convince consumers to buy their products (*How can advertisements influence your food choices?*, 2020). Some of the strategies they use to convince us include:

- Making health or nutrient claims, e.g., calcium builds strong bones. You'll often see these claims on dairy and calcium-enriched products. While calcium is a major component of our skeletons, these claims are technically a half-truth. Calcium alone is not enough to ensure strong, healthy bones. Our bodies need other nutrients to absorb and make use of calcium.
- Bright colors, freebies, celebrity spokespeople, discount prices and catchy jingles and catchphrases are all part of the usual marketing gamut.

Advertisements are designed to make certain foods appear more desirable, potentially shaping beliefs and attitudes toward food. This can happen through:

- **Product promotion:** Advertising and marketing can be used to promote certain foods, making them appear more desirable and appealing to consumers. For example, an advertisement for a fast-food burger may make it seem more delicious and satisfying than it is.
- **Brand loyalty:** Advertising and marketing can be used to create brand loyalty, which can make it more likely for consumers to choose certain foods over others. For example, suppose a

person is exposed to a lot of advertising for a particular cereal brand. In that case, they may be more likely to choose that cereal over other brands, even if healthier options are available.

- **Misinformation:** Advertising and marketing can be used to spread misinformation about food, nutrition, and health claims. This can be done through deceptive or misleading advertising or using scientific-sounding terms and buzzwords without scientific support. For example, "all-natural" claims on a food product don't have a standard definition and are not regulated by the FDA, so these claims may be misleading.

- **Targeting specific groups:** Advertisements and marketing can target specific groups, such as children, low-income communities, or older adults, and can influence the food choices of these groups. For example, a cereal company may target advertising to children to create brand loyalty and influence their food choices as they grow older.

- **Diet culture reinforcement:** Advertisements and marketing can reinforce diet culture messages, prioritizing weight loss, thinness, and control over food, and pressuring individuals to conform to a specific body type and size.

Becoming aware of the tactics that food advertisers employ can help protect you from unhealthy food choices. Recent research found that teenagers are especially vulnerable to food marketing. Ads targeting teenagers typically promote highly processed foods, and there's a reason for that. A lot of teenagers' decision-making is influenced by their peers, and food companies have simply tapped into it (and social media) to drive their food choices (David, 2020).

It's no wonder then that we are seeing an increasing number of teenagers and young children becoming obese. According to the CDC, nearly a quarter (20.6%) of teens between the ages of 12 and 19 are obese (*Childhood obesity facts,* 2022). Obesity at any age is strongly linked to a multitude of health problems.

HEALTH CONCERNS ABOUT THE IMPACT OF FOOD CHOICE

For general health and wellbeing, a good diet is essential. However, it's critical to keep in mind that eating a "good" diet might raise certain health issues, particularly if the diet is restricted, imbalanced, or founded on false information. People with health concerns, such as diabetes or heart disease, may make different food choices than those without these concerns. They often choose foods to help them manage their condition and follow dietary recommendations. When it comes to health concerns, it is pertinent to keep the following in mind:

- **Nutrient deficiencies:** An overly restrictive diet or eliminating entire food groups can lead to nutrient deficiencies. This can occur if a person does not consume enough specific vitamins, minerals, or other essential nutrients. For example, a vegetarian diet that doesn't include dairy, eggs, or fortified plant-based alternatives may lead to a deficiency in Vitamin B12, a vital nutrient for the proper functioning of the brain and nervous system.
- **Disordered eating:** Restrictive dieting and an obsession with weight loss can lead to disordered eating patterns, such as binge eating, overeating, or fasting. These patterns can harm physical and emotional well-being and lead to severe eating disorders.
- **Impact on mental health:** Dieting can increase the risk of developing depression, anxiety, and low self-esteem, as well as cognitive distortions about food and weight (Muhlheim, 2017). Before making major dietary changes, develop a healthy relationship with food first.

- **Burden on lifestyle:** Eating a restrictive diet can become an all-consuming task. It can make it challenging to participate in social activities or enjoy eating out, leading to isolation and stress. For example, individuals who have a ketogenic diet need to avoid sugars and starches. A lot of our food items at social gatherings contain sugars and starches in some form, so it becomes difficult for these individuals to fully participate. They may become isolated as a result of their dietary choices as it is very difficult in our modern food landscape to avoid sugars and starches all together.

- **Negative impact on metabolism:** Eating too few calories and too little variety of foods can negatively affect the metabolism, which, in the long term, can result in weight gain and decreased health. When we lower our food intake dramatically the body goes into "starvation mode" and assumes food is scarce (Spritzler, 2019). In this state our metabolism slows down since the body is trying to hold on to energy reserves as long as possible. It is a survival mechanism that served our ancestors well but is doing modern man with abundant food supplies no favors.

The outcome of the seven factors that influence food choices is that they all interact and contribute to an individual's overall dietary habits and preferences. These factors can work together to shape a person's eating patterns and can affect their risk for diet-related health issues such as obesity, heart disease, and diabetes. They can also impact an individual's ability to access healthy food options, affecting their overall health and well-being. It is essential to understand how these factors interact and affect food choices in order to make informed decisions about one's diet and improve overall health. The activity below is designed to help guide you on your journey to make informed food choices.

FOOD DIARY-BASED ACTION

Food diaries are useful tools that help us keep track of our eating habits. There are numerous reasons why we would keep a food diary. These reasons range from weight management to improving our overall health. Food diaries are valuable tools that can help your healthcare provider understand your eating habits, but more importantly, these diaries can help us evaluate our relationship with food in a healthy way. The diary below is designed to help us reconnect with our hunger and satiety cues. By assigning a number to how hungry

or satiated we are (1 being extremely hungry/not satiated and 10 being not hungry/very full), it becomes
much easier to recognize these cues. Numerical values
also make it easy to spot trends, for example, if certain
meals leave you feeling stuffed or unsatisfied.

Meal	How Hungry I Felt (scored from 1–10)	Food Consumed	Amount Consumed	How Satiated I Felt (scored from 1–10)	Notes
Breakfast	4	Cereal with milk and orange juice.	One cup of cereal. Half a cup of whole milk. One glass of orange juice.	8	Cereal kept me feeling full for a short while, but I became very hungry before lunch time.
Lunch	2	Pasta alfredo and iced tea.	One serving of pasta (prepared by restaurant). Two glasses of iced tea (prepared by restaurant).	10	I felt very full and sluggish after the meal.
Dinner	7	An apple, nuts and cranberry juice.	One large apple. A quarter cup of unsalted nuts. One glass of cranberry juice.	9	I still felt very full after lunch and had some snacks instead.

Breakfast					
Lunch					
Dinner					

2

PSYCHOLOGICAL FACTORS OF EATING HEALTHY

Several psychological factors influence our food choices. Genetics, culture, and early experiences with food can all affect these preferences, but our emotions affect food choices as well. Some people eat certain foods to cope with stress. These emotional eating habits can lead to overeating and harm overall health.

Food choices are also affected by memory. People associate certain foods with positive memories, such as the taste of a dish that reminds them of a favorite childhood restaurant. The emotional connection with particular foods can lead to cravings. Over time, these factors can change. An individual's taste preference may change, or an emotional relationship to certain foods may vary due to life circumstances. The psychological factors interact with other factors that influence food choices. Sometimes our strongest food cravings surface when we are at a low point in our lives. We might find ourselves turning to food, either consciously or unconsciously, as a source of comfort or as a way to deal with stress (*Weight loss: gain control of emotional eating*, 2022). Emotional eating and comfort foods can derail our efforts to eat healthy, which makes it extra important to understand the psychological aspects of eating.

Eating healthy is not just about the physical aspects of food but also the psychological factors that influence our food choices. The psychology of eating healthy refers to how our thoughts, emotions, and behaviors affect our food choices and eating habits. It encompasses a range of factors that can influence our decisions about what to eat, including our motivation, self-control, stress levels, social influences, mindfulness, perceptions and beliefs, emotions and moods, and self-esteem. Understanding these psychological factors can help us make better food choices and maintain a healthy lifestyle. We will explore the psychological factors that influence our eating habits and how to use them to make healthier food choices.

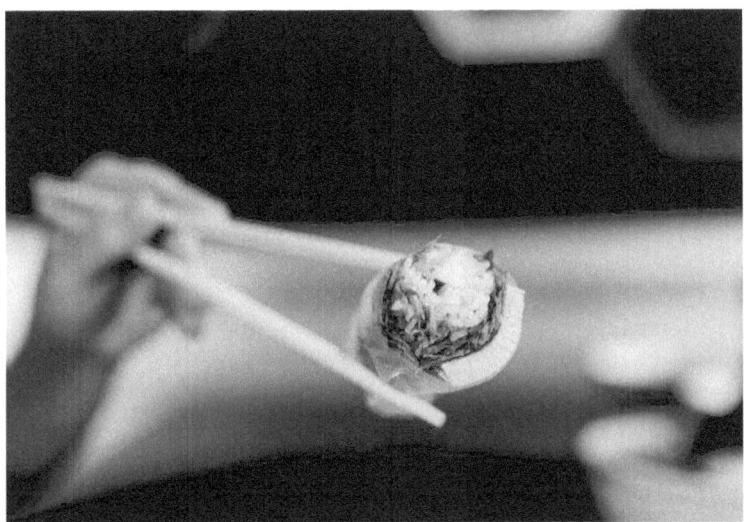

TASTE PREFERENCES

People prefer certain types of food, such as sweet, salty, or spicy. These preferences are often developed early in life, but many factors can influence them. Culture, family, past experiences, and exposure to different flavors are some of the important factors that influence how our taste preferences develop.

- **Genetics:**

Studies have shown that particular taste preferences, such as a preference for sweet or bitter foods, are influenced by genetics. One way genetics influence our taste is by determining how intensely our taste buds can perceive certain tastes, as is the case with bitter compounds (Moller, 2021). Sweet and bitter tastes largely determine which foods we enjoy and which ones we reject. Not surprisingly, most people (especially infants) seem to prefer a sweeter taste. This could be due to a genetic predisposition. Our genes, specifically a variant of the ALDH2 gene, are strongly linked with the preference for sweet tastes (Kawafune et al., 2020).

So, some people's sweet tooth can be attributed to genetics, at least in part. It is believed that our preference for sweet tastes is due to an evolutionary adaptation that encouraged early man to consume energy-rich foods (Wilson, 2022). While some of our taste preferences can be explained by genetics, it does not provide the full picture, and a lot of research is still needed to establish how genetics influence our taste preferences.

- **Past experiences:**

Previous experiences with certain foods, such as childhood experiences or cultural background, can shape taste preferences. The idea of eating chicken feet may sound off-putting to some, but for those who grew up in South Africa, South America, East Asia, and the Caribbean, this dish is part of the normal fare. The foods we were exposed to growing up greatly influences our taste preferences later in life. It should be noted that taste preferences are not set in stone and can change.

I'll share a little secret with you: I hated spinach well into my 20s due to a past experience. When I was young, my parents maintained an organic vegetable patch. That means no pesticides or chemical fertilizer were used, and the veggies tasted great. It also meant insects would inevitably make a home in those luscious spinach bunches. Even though the spinach was thoroughly washed before being cooked, one of those beautifully camouflaged green bugs managed to evade detection. It ended up on my plate and my eight-year-old self took a hearty bite out of the bitter creature. It took many years and a lot of coaxing before I tried spinach again. It didn't matter to me if it was home-grown or store bought; in my mind, that bitter green bug was still hiding in those spinach bunches. Many years later, I rediscovered my love for spinach, but it just goes to show that our experiences with food greatly influence how willing we are to eat it again in the future.

- **Environmental factors:**

Exposure to different foods, flavors, and food preparation methods can influence taste preferences. Take sushi as an example. Authentic Japanese sushi and the versions we find in America are very different. One would assume that rice, seafood, and seaweed would have a pretty standard taste, but this is not the case. Regional tastes and cultural differences have had a big influence on how sushi is prepared and presented in other parts of the world (Ransom, 2017). For example, Western diners may prefer bright colors and bold flavors, which explains why the Philadelphia Roll is so popular. It is usually prepared with salmon, avocado, and cream cheese. In Japan, sushi is prepared to reflect a delicate balance of flavors. There are many variants that reflect the local taste preferences and ingredients.

- **Psychological and emotional factors:**

Emotions and moods can also influence taste preferences. For example, stress or anxiety may lead to cravings for high-fat or high-sugar foods. We may feel the need to respond to high-intensity emotions like stress, anxiety, sadness, anger and happiness by eating comfort foods. While these foods provide a brief feeling of comfort, eating our emotions can lead to long-term unresolved issues and negative health consequences (Sheth, 2023). It is easy to reach for and finish that bag of chips or tub of ice cream when we are in an emotional state, but doing so can place a serious stick in one's spokes.

Emotional eating can set the stage for eating disorders and food addictions. Fortunately, there is help available for individuals who find themselves trapped in the cycle of emotional eating. Stress management, community support, and therapy (in some cases) can go a long way toward helping us regain control of our emotions and eating habits. We'll explore how emotions impact our eating habits in more detail in a separate section.

- **Nutritional status:**

A person's nutritional status can also affect taste preferences. For example, a deficiency in vitamin B12 and zinc are associated with a loss in taste, but this can normally be reversed through a healthy diet and supplements (*Dysgeusia*, n.d.).

- **Health conditions:**

Certain medical conditions, such as diabetes or heart disease, may require changes in diet that may not align with one's taste preferences. Illnesses and accidents can drastically alter our taste perception. Conditions like Alzheimer's, dementia, and cancer are known to drastically influence taste perception (*10 surprising factors that affect your taste perception*, n.d.). A combination of illness and medical treatment can sometimes completely alter our sense of taste.

EMOTIONS IMPACT YOUR FOOD CHOICES

Turning to food for comfort in order to cope with difficult or big feelings is quite common. According to the American Psychological Association, 33% of adults who turn to food due to stress do so because it is a form of distraction (*Stress and eating*, 2013). More worrisome still is that this behavior is often a habit. Food can evoke strong emotional responses. As a result, people may choose to indulge in foods they associate with positive emotions, such as comfort or happiness. Additionally, people may use food to cope with difficult emotions. Some of the reasons why people turn to food for comfort include:

- **Stress:** Stress can lead to emotional eating, which can result in overeating or choosing unhealthy foods as a coping mechanism.
- **Anxiety:** Anxiety can cause changes in appetite and lead to emotional eating.
- **Depression:** Depression can lead to changes in appetite and a lack of interest in food, resulting in poor nutrition.

- **Boredom:** Boredom can lead to emotional eating and the consumption of high-calorie foods as a form of entertainment.
- **Lack of control:** A lack of control in one's life can lead to emotional eating as a form of self-soothing.
- **Social pressure:** Social pressure can lead to overeating or consuming certain foods in social situations.
- **Trauma:** Trauma can lead to emotional eating as a coping mechanism.

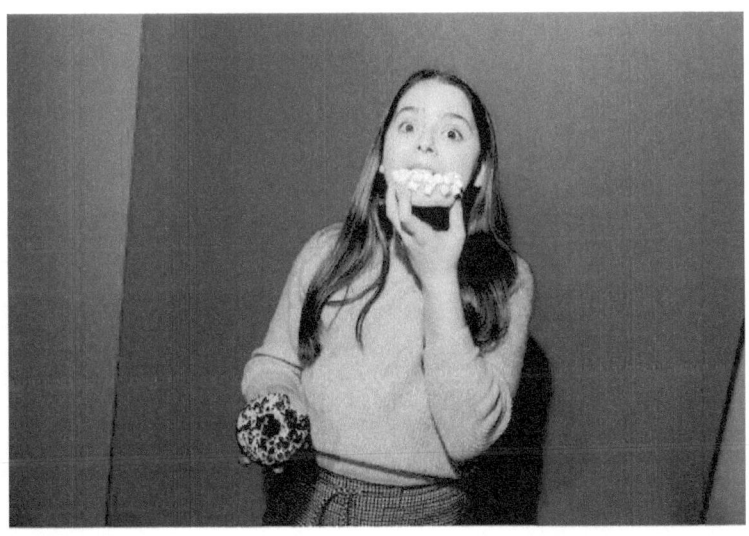

Anytime we eat in response to an emotion, it is considered emotional eating. Whether we grab an ice cream to "celebrate" good news or turn to that bag of cookies to get over a breakup, know that everyone does this sometimes. It is when emotional eating happens frequently and we don't have other ways to cope with difficult emotions that it can become a serious problem.

Food lights up our bodies' reward system, making us feel better. So in the moment, it may feel like a way of coping with challenging emotions and situations (Marcin, 2018). However, in the long run, eating to cope with difficult situations and emotions is like sticking a Band-Aid on a bullet wound. No amount of food can fix stress, anxiety, trauma, or boredom. Worse still, emotional eating can lead to feelings of guilt and shame in some individuals. This creates more difficult feelings that can trigger the craving for comfort food.

MEMORY OF FOOD

Our memories of past experiences with food can also influence our food choices. People may choose foods that they associate with positive memories, such as a favorite childhood dish, or avoid foods that they associate with negative experiences (like the bug in my spinach experience). Some of the factors impacting our memory of food include:

- **Food associations:** Positive memories associated with certain foods can make a person more likely to choose those foods, even if they are unhealthy. For example, if a person has fond memories of eating ice cream with their family as a child, they may be more likely to choose it as a treat, even if it is unhealthy.
- **Eating habits:** Past experiences with food can also shape a person's eating habits. For example, if a person has negative memories associated with eating healthy foods, they may be less likely to choose those foods in the present.
- **Emotional eating:** People may use food as a coping mechanism for emotional issues, and memories of past traumas or events can trigger emotional eating.
- **Social cues:** Memories of past social experiences with food can influence the food choices a person makes in the present. For example, if a person has fond memories of eating a certain dish with friends or family, they may be more likely to choose it when eating with those people.

Food is at the center of many human activities. Examining our food memories can help us take control of our eating patterns.

FOOD NEOPHOBIA

Some people fear trying new foods, a phenomenon known as food neophobia. People with this condition tend to stick to familiar foods and may avoid new or unfamiliar foods, which can limit their food choices. One of the most famous and extreme cases of food neophobia is that of Austin Davis. The Florida resident openly spoke on *VICE* and *LADbible* about his preference for macaroni and cheese, claiming that it was the only food he ate for nearly two decades (Florida man only eats mac and cheese for last 17 years, 2023)! Davis' food neophobia is sadly fueled by a severe anxiety disorder called Avoidant/Restrictive Food Intake Disorder (AFRID). People with this condition might avoid certain foods or food groups due to the texture, smell, taste, or appearance thereof (*ARFID*, n.d.). Some of the factors that characterize food neophobia include the following:

- **Limited food choices:** People with food neophobia may limit their food choices to familiar foods, making it difficult to eat a balanced and varied diet. This may lead to nutrient deficiencies and a lack of exposure to new flavors and textures.

- **Poor nutrition:** Food neophobia can make it difficult for people to try new foods that are healthy or beneficial for their diet. This may lead to a lack of nutrients and may increase the risk of chronic disease.
- **Social limitations:** Food neophobia can also affect social interactions and make it difficult for people to participate in meals with friends and family.
- **Impacts children:** Children with food neophobia may be at risk for malnutrition, poor growth and development, and may have a limited diet.

Several strategies can help individuals overcome food neophobia, including exposure therapy, cognitive-behavioral therapy, and education about the benefits of healthy foods. It is also important to expose children to new foods early, to help them develop a positive relationship with food and a willingness to try new things.

It is important to note that food neophobia is not always bad, as some people may be picky eaters because they have food allergies or sensitivities that they are aware of. Some may have strong cultural or personal reasons for not eating certain foods.

OBESITY AFFECTS FOOD CHOICE

Obesity can be a psychological condition as well. People who are overweight or obese may have difficulty sticking to a healthy diet due to emotional factors such as self-esteem, depression, and body image concerns. Other factors influencing obesity need to be considered, and this includes:

- **Physical limitations:**

Obesity can make it difficult for individuals to engage in physical activity, making it harder to maintain a healthy weight. People with obesity may also experience physical discomfort or pain when engaging in physical activity, which can make it less appealing. Exercises that place minimal stress on the joints, like swimming and walking, are recommended as a good starting point for most individuals who want to become physically active.

- **Emotional and psychological factors:**

Obesity can also significantly impact a person's emotional and psychological well-being. People with obesity may experience shame, self-esteem issues, and body dissatisfaction, making it difficult to engage in healthy eating behaviors. These emotions can trigger emotional eating and other unhealthy coping mechanisms which makes it harder to maintain a healthy weight.

- **Food choices:**

Obesity can also affect a person's food choices. People who are overweight may be more likely to choose high-calorie, high-fat foods that are less nutritious. Despite the ease of access to food that most people have, very few of us are given a proper food education. Nutrition education is essential, especially when we are looking to make lasting and healthy lifestyle changes.

- **Access to healthy food:**

People with obesity may also have limited access to healthy food options due to economic, social, or geographic factors.

- **Metabolic factors:**

Obesity can also lead to metabolic issues, making it harder for people to lose weight and maintain a healthy diet. For example, people with obesity may have difficulty regulating their blood sugar levels, which can make it harder to control cravings for unhealthy foods. The metabolic complications that come with obesity often include insulin resistance, hypertension, and sleep apnea (Singla, 2010).

Overall, obesity can make it more challenging to engage in healthy eating behaviors, but it is not impossible.

Our food choices are influenced by a complex interplay of psychological, emotional, and memory-related factors that can make it challenging to make healthy food choices. Understanding these factors can help us develop strategies to overcome them and make healthier food choices.

FOOD DIARY-BASED ACTION

We are going to add a little bit more to the food diary we started developing in Chapter 1. This food diary activity is designed to help us recognize emotional eating patterns. In Chapter 1's food diary activity, the goal was to reconnect with the body's hunger and satiety signals. In this activity, we will still score our hunger and satiety levels from 1–10 like we did in the last chapter, but we are going to reflect on whether our emotions triggered our eating. When you write your diary entry, ask yourself the following:

- Did I experience strong emotions before my meal? If so, what triggered these emotions?
- Did I eat to cope with my emotions or stress?
- How did I feel after the meal?

Meal	How Hungry I Felt (scored from 1–10)	Food Consumed	Amount Consumed	How Satiated I Felt (scored from 1–10)	Did I Eat My Emotions? How did I feel afterwards?
Breakfast	2	English breakfast and coffee.	Traditional English breakfast with eggs, sausage, and bacon (prepared by a restaurant). One cup of coffee with sugar and milk (prepared by a restaurant).	10	I was very upset and stressed about the fight I had with my partner last night. I still felt upset after the meal.
Lunch	7	Slice of cake and milkshake.	One slice of chocolate cake and a thick, strawberry milkshake (prepared by a restaurant).	10	I felt very full and very sluggish. I still felt upset about the fight and ate even though I was not hungry.
Dinner	7	Juice	Four glasses of orange juice.	9	I did not feel hungry and skipped dinner. I only had some juice. I didn't feel so upset about the fight anymore.

Breakfast					
Lunch					
Dinner					

3

HOW DIET CULTURE PUTS MORE PRESSURE

Our media and daily lives are saturated with examples of diet culture. Sometimes these examples are overt and easy to spot, such as an ad for "detox tea" on your social media feed or a friend touting the virtues of a crash diet. Sometimes the sneakiness of diet culture is more difficult to detect. But what exactly is "diet culture"?

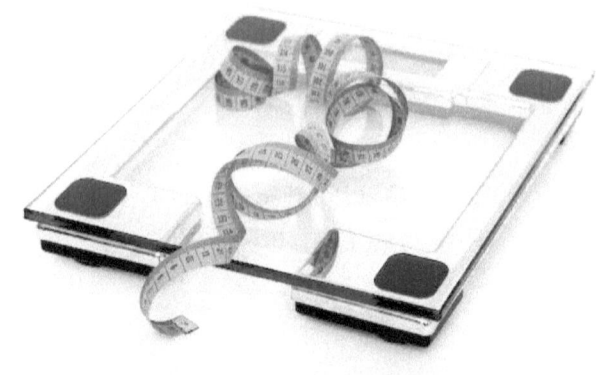

Diet culture refers to societal and cultural beliefs and practices prioritizing weight loss, thinness, and the pursuit of a particular body shape or size. This belief takes priority over our overall health and well-being. It encompasses a set of beliefs and values that promote weight loss, certain types of food as "good" or "bad," and value thinness over health. Diet culture can be harmful and lead to disordered eating and body image issues. It can also perpetuate weight stigma and discrimination. When we look at diet culture as a whole, it certainly does not promote a healthy relationship with food or our bodies.

Diet culture is not a new phenomenon. We can thank the ancient Greeks for the earliest known incarnation of it. Ancient Greeks promoted the idea of moderating and regulating food intake as a way to promote self-control, one of the highest virtues in ancient Greek culture (*Diet culture throughout history*, 2022). Controlling food intake was a means to attain health and a balanced body, which the ancient Greeks considered to be aesthetically pleasing.

Diet culture has been around for a long time but has evolved and changed over the years. The origins of diet culture can be traced back to the 19th century, when the term "diet" was first used to refer to the food and drink a person consumed. In the early 20th century, diet culture was associated with weight loss and the idea that thinner was better.

In the 1950s and 1960s, diet culture began to be heavily promoted by the diet and weight-loss industries. This was when weight loss products, diet books, and weight loss programs became more prevalent. Diet culture was also influenced by societal expectations, with thinness considered the ideal body type. In the 1980s and 1990s, diet culture became more mainstream with the rise of diet fads and the promotion of restrictive and unrealistic diet plans.

The media also heavily influenced diet culture, with certain body types and sizes portrayed as ideal. Shows like *The Biggest Loser* and self-proclaimed fitness gurus frequently judged people based on how vigorously they exercised and how religiously they adhered to a restrictive (if not oppressive) diet. Keep in mind that these are people that the shows and gurus were supposed to help. A quick web search into *The Biggest Loser's* success rate shows that, on average, the participants regained 70% of the weight they had lost within 6 years (Fothergill et al., 2016). This just goes to show that the extreme form of diet culture and fitness obsession promoted by the media is unhelpful and unsustainable for a healthy body in the long run.

In recent years, diet culture has become more pervasive with the rise of social media and the proliferation of diet and fitness influencers. Social media and our assumption that thinness is linked to a healthy body created the perfect environment for toxic food and fitness myths to spread—all for the sake of gaining more followers. Hannah Berry, a fitness influencer based in the United Kingdom, took to social media, revealing the unsavory tactics influencers resort to. One of these questionable tactics includes the promotion of smoothies, drinks, teas, cleanses, or detox programs to "balance hormones" (Mather, 2023). Berry also revealed that other fitness influencers would offer to buy her transformation photos. They wanted these photos to sell their fitness program, tricking followers into thinking that the program was effective.

Whether it is "body checking" on TikTok or the "thigh gap" trend on Tumblr, the media, societal expectations, the diet and fitness industry, and social media all have a hand in perpetuating diet culture. Knowing the red flags of diet culture can help us avoid falling victim to oppressive ideals and unscrupulous influencers. We'll examine these red flags a bit closer in the content that follows.

SOCIETAL PRESSURE

It is reinforced by societal messages prioritizing thinness and promoting unrealistic body standards. These messages do not take into account that we are all unique individuals with a unique set of circumstances. Conforming to these ideals can cause stress and lead to feelings of inadequacy and low self-esteem in individuals. There are many ways these messages of unrealistic body standards are communicated, including:

- **Media representation:**

The media often promotes certain body types and shapes as the ideal, which can pressure individuals to conform to these standards. This can lead people to try fad diets, restrictive eating patterns, and other harmful behaviors, such as Gwyneth Paltrow's "elimination diet." Celebrities are often represented in the media as an embodiment of beauty ideals (Brown & Tiggemann, 2021). When we consider that the predominant cultural ideal (especially for women) is thinness, the constant media exposure to these ideas can trigger a deep-seated dissatisfaction with our bodies. Body dissatisfaction can have severe negative effects on our mental and physical health and can lead to the development of depression and eating disorders.

- **Healthism:**

Healthism is the belief that health is a moral imperative and an individual's worth is based on health. This belief can contribute to societal pressure to conform to specific health standards, even if it is unhealthy for an individual. An extreme incarnation of healthism is orthorexia. It is defined as having an obsession with eating healthy foods in order to avoid poor health (Hui, 2022). It is not clear what causes orthorexia, but researchers believe a history of disordered eating and poor body image contribute toward it. Some signs of orthorexia include cutting out entire food groups, constantly checking nutrition fact labels, becoming distressed when healthy foods are not available and obsessively following food health blogs and news.

- **Beauty standards:**

Societal pressure to conform to specific beauty standards can lead people to believe that they must conform to certain body types to be considered attractive or desirable.

- **Economic factors:**

Societal pressure can also come from economic factors, such as the weight loss industry, that profits from people's insecurities and desire to conform to certain body standards.

Society often promotes the idea that thinner is better and that certain body types are more desirable than others. This can create pressure to conform to these ideals, leading to disordered eating patterns and body image issues. In the long run, these messages do not promote a healthy relationship with food or our bodies. Instead, we may end up treating food as the enemy and our bodies as a battleground.

CONSTANT MESSAGING

Diet culture is often marketed and promoted through various media outlets and products. This often leads to continuous messaging about weight loss, dieting, and body ideals. This can put you under constant pressure to diet and work toward weight loss. Some of the ways these messages are disseminated include:

- **Marketing and advertising:** The food and weight loss industries heavily advertise their products and services, which can create a constant stream of messaging about dieting and weight loss.
- **Social media:** Social media platforms are often used to promote diet culture, with influencers and celebrities sharing diet tips, weight loss transformations, and promoting restrictive eating patterns.
- **Health and wellness industry:** The health and wellness industry can also contribute to the constant messaging of diet culture by promoting specific diets or supplements as the solution to health problems.
- **Celebrity culture:** Celebrity culture can contribute to the constant messaging of diet culture by promoting the idea that certain body types are desirable or attainable.
- **Media interpretation:** The media can contribute to the constant messaging of diet culture by promoting certain body types and

shapes as the ideal and focusing on weight loss and dieting as a means to achieve that ideal.

The constant messaging of diet culture can make it difficult for people to understand what healthy eating truly is. It can also create a sense of guilt and shame for people who do not conform to these standards and can lead to disordered eating patterns.

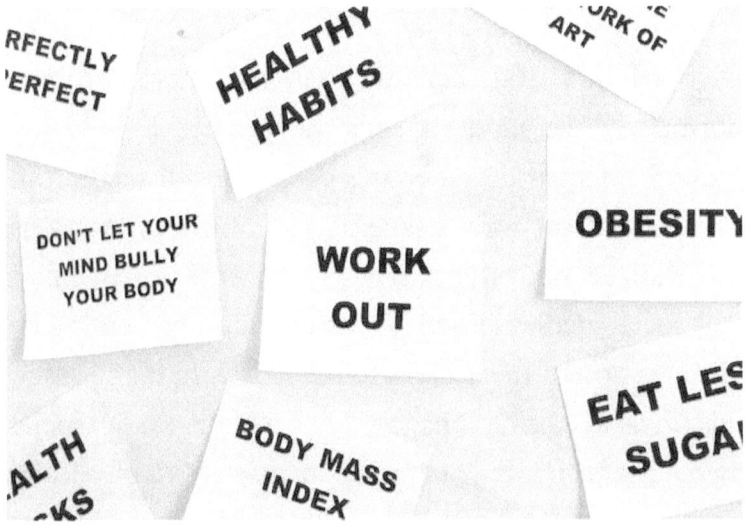

EMPHASIS ON CONTROL

Social media can also contribute to diet culture by promoting the idea that weight loss and thinness are necessary for happiness, health, and success. This can create pressure to conform to certain ideals, leading to disordered eating patterns and body image issues. Additionally, diet culture normalizes negative self-talk (Daryanani, 2021). Examples of negative self-talk include:

- My arms are too flabby.
- That ice cream has too many calories.
- I'll get fat if I eat this.
- After that slice of cake, I'm going to the gym.

Diet culture and negative self-talk have become normalized in modern society, creating a breeding ground for disordered eating habits. Social media can adversely affect body image by constantly exposing us to idealized body types (Heger, 2022). Keep in mind that social media is filled with individuals presenting an ideal version of themselves to the world. In many cases, this means editing images. As a result, many social media users end up comparing themselves to physically unachievable and unrealistic images, which further drives body dissatisfaction.

Notably, researchers found that the majority of social media users edit their images in some way. Nearly 70% of women and 50% of men between the ages of 18 and 35 reported that they regularly edited their images (Guest, 2016). These findings speak of a widespread dissatisfaction with our natural bodies, to the point where presenting an edited ideal seems normal.

Social media can also contribute to the emphasis on control by promoting restrictive eating patterns and showcasing people who have achieved significant weight loss through strict control over their food choices. This emphasis on control can lead to disordered eating patterns such as orthorexia, an obsession with eating only "pure" or "healthy" foods, and anorexia, an eating disorder characterized by low weight, a fear of weight gain, and a distorted body image. It can also lead to guilt and shame when individuals cannot exert control over their food choices and body weight. It is important to remember that health is not just about physical appearance but also mental and emotional well-being.

There are some simple steps we can take to protect ourselves from the toxic diet culture on our social media feeds. These steps include:

- Avoiding negative self-talk.
- Embrace and celebrate your natural self by refusing to edit photos.
- Realize that being thin does not mean you are healthy.

- Models, influencers and celebrities are not representative of the average person's body. Don't compare yourself to them.
- Clean up your feed by unfollowing toxic accounts that promote the "ideal" body.

A healthy relationship with food starts by accepting your natural body. Remember, you are beautiful and worthy, no matter what the scale or influencer says!

FOOD RESTRICTION

The weight-loss services industry is a lucrative market, with the U.S. market valued at nearly four billion dollars (*Weight loss services in the US: market size 2003–2028*, 2022). We know from research that fad diets are not an effective means of weight management in the long run—a truth that is harshly reflected in the healthy bottom line of the weight management industry. This industry is so profitable because it feeds into the vicious cycle that diet culture sets in motion, i.e., the belief that our natural bodies are not good enough and that we need to "fix" them somehow. This toxic foundation of diet culture sets the individual up to treat their body as a problem, which creates a lucrative industry in a capitalist society. A quick glance at all the diet products in the drugstore and online is evidence enough of this.

If questionable teas, tonics, pills, and patches were our only concern, then perhaps the weight loss industry would not be so pervasive. As it stands, the lines between nutrition and blatant misinformation are often blurred, encouraging consumers to restrict their intake of certain foods. Tips such as "eat this" or "don't eat that" perpetuate the idea that certain foods are inherently bad. Usually, it is dietary fat that is labeled as "bad," but it depends on the trending diet. Some diets, like the "ketogenic lifestyle," encourage individuals to cut out carbs and sugars entirely. Most fruits and vegetables are sources of dietary carbs and sugars, so you can imagine how restrictive it would be to eat in a ketogenic way. There are individuals that need to eat like this for medical reasons, but many who jump on the keto bandwagon do so for weight-loss purposes.

Other diets encourage individuals to cut out as much fat as possible. These diets do not take into account that our bodies need various food sources to stay healthy. Dietary fats, for example, help with the absorption of vitamins A, D, E, and K—all fat-soluble vitamins, whereas fruits and vegetables are rich sources of vitamins and minerals. To eliminate an entire food group from our diets, whether it be fats, carbs, protein in the form of meat, or the sugars found in fruit, is simply a recipe for ill-health.

Demonizing certain food groups can encourage a very rigid way of thinking about food and our bodies, leading to extreme approaches to weight loss if the outcome we want is not achieved. This is when individuals can easily fall prey to fad diets like an "elimination diet" or questionable weight loss products to achieve the weight they desire.

The diet and fitness industries can create pressure by promoting restrictive and unrealistic diet plans and workout routines, leading to disordered eating patterns and body image issues. Promoting restrictive eating behaviors and eliminating certain foods or food groups can pressurize us to eliminate certain food groups, but there's a psychological aspect to it as well. When we fail to adhere to an impossibly restrictive diet it can lead to feelings of guilt and shame when indulging in certain foods. If we are honest and realistic, we'd realize that human beings love flavor and variety. Nobody would want to stay stuck on an oppressive diet of steamed chicken and cruciferous vegetables! Variety is the spice of life, and these fad diets are essentially designed for failure. When one diet doesn't work for us, we try another and then another.

Food restriction can lead to nutrient deficiencies and can also create a preoccupation with food and a fear of certain foods, known as food phobia. These phobias can make it difficult for individuals to enjoy meals and socialize. It can also lead to eating disorders such as anorexia, which is characterized by low weight, a fear of gaining weight, and a distorted body image.

PRESSURE ON PHYSICAL APPEARANCE

Friends and family members may also contribute to diet culture by commenting on weight, dieting, or appearance, which can create pressure to conform to certain ideals. This situation is often exacerbated when we have poor body image.

"Body image" refers to how we think and feel about our bodies (*Body image and diets*, 2013). What we feel and think about our bodies is not necessarily a true reflection of what we see in the mirror. Poor body image is often characterized by:

- over-exercising.
- dieting.
- disordered eating such as anorexia nervosa, orthorexia, binge eating, or bulimia nervosa.
- mental health issues like depression, low self-esteem, or anxiety.

Poor body image can also arise from comparing our bodies with representations of the "ideal" body in the media. Keep in mind that this ideal varies over time and between cultures. According to research, some women who moved to Australia developed different eating habits and body images as they adapted to their new environment (Babatunde-Sowole et al., 2018). This shows us that body image and diet habits are fluid concepts that can change to accommodate our surroundings.

Our social circle can place a lot of emphasis on the importance of physical appearance and body weight. This can create pressure to conform to specific physical standards, which can lead to low self-esteem and other difficult emotions. It is important to remember that beauty and health come in all different shapes and sizes. The world would indeed be dreadfully dull if we all looked like copy-and-paste versions of each other! The important thing is that individuals strive to make choices that are best for their health and well-being rather than conforming to societal norms and expectations.

FOCUS ON A QUICK FIX

Promises of quick and easy solutions for weight loss run rampant in diet culture. This can create pressure to find the perfect diet and lead to feelings of failure when those promises do not come to fruition. Diet culture promotes the idea that weight loss can be achieved through quick and easy solutions, such as fad diets, restrictive eating patterns, and supplements. These misleading ideas are often propagated through various channels, including:

- **Media representation:**

The media often promotes quick-fix diet and weight loss solutions, such as juice cleanses, detox teas, and other products that promise rapid weight loss. The products commonly have undesirable side-effects and can be dangerous in some cases. Detox teas, for example, are known to cause abdominal pain, bloating, gas, and nausea (Cirino, 2019). These side effects are still benign when compared to other, potentially dangerous, products on the market. Certain "diet pills" are linked to an increased risk of lung, colorectal, and pancreatic cancer (Poteet, 2021).

- **Social media:**

Influencers in your feed can add pressure by focusing on quick-fix solutions and promoting other influencers and celebrities who have achieved significant weight loss through restrictive diets and supplements. As we discovered early in this chapter, the influencer world is hardly a clean-cut one and these individuals may resort to questionable tactics for the sake of gaining more followers. Hannah Berry's confession clearly points this out. Keep in mind that not all fitness influencers fall into this toxic camp, but we need to be extra careful about who we follow on social media.

- **Economic factors:**

Weight loss, fitness, and other related industries can contribute to the pressure to focus on quick-fix solutions by profiting from people's desire to lose weight quickly.

- **Healthism:**

This belief can contribute to the pressure to focus on quick-fix solutions by promoting the idea that weight loss and good health can be achieved quickly and easily.

Society's pressure to focus on quick-fix solutions can lead to unrealistic expectations, disappointment, and negative mental and physical health effects. It is critical to remember that weight loss and healthy eating are long-term commitments and that professional assistance should be sought when necessary.

It's essential to remember that diet culture is not the only means to being healthy. Weight loss is not necessary for health, nor is it a one-size-fits-all solution to everyone's health and well-being challenges. Diet culture can be harmful and can lead to eating disorders, body dissatisfaction, and other challenges. It is critical to prioritize overall health and well-being over weight loss or a specific body shape. Developing a healthy relationship with food and your body is key. It's important to note that diet culture has evolved and will continue to do so as new trends and technologies emerge.

FOOD DIARY-BASED ACTION

The way we perceive our bodies plays a big role in how susceptible we are to diet culture. This food-diary entry is designed to help you become more aware of how you perceive your body. When we have a deeper understanding of how we view our bodies, it is possible to make strides on the road to healthy living without falling victim to harmful diet culture messages. We'll take note of our hunger, satiety levels, and emotions just like we did in the previous chapter, but we'll add one extra element: An assessment of how we feel about our bodies. When assessing how we feel about our bodies, reflect on the following questions:

- How do you feel about yourself and your body today?
- Take a look at your reflection. Do you like what you see? Elaborate on your answer.
- How comfortable do you feel in your skin today? Elaborate on your answer.

Meal	How Hungry I Felt (scored from 1–10)	Food Consumed	Amount Consumed	How Satiated I Felt (scored from 1–10)	Did I Eat My Emotions? How did I feel afterwards?
Breakfast	3	Oats and juice.	One serving of oats (prepared myself) with a glass of orange juice.	8	I ate because I was hungry.
Lunch	5	Burger, fries, and a milkshake.	One chicken burger, sweet potato fries and a strawberry milkshake (prepared by restaurant)	10	I felt upset after a coworker made a remark about my body. I ate too much and felt sluggish.
Dinner	5	Fish, vegetables, and water.	Steamed fish, broccoli, and carrots (prepared at home).	9	My coworker's comment is still bothering me, so I'm trying to eat extra healthy to feel better.

How Do I Feel About My Body Today? Why?					
Today I felt a bit uncomfortable in my own skin. A coworker made a comment about my body that made me feel self-conscious. The comment bothered me so much that I went for an extra-long walk this evening. I felt better after the walk.					
Breakfast					
Lunch					
Dinner					

How Do I Feel About My Body Today? Why?

4

AWARENESS OF BIOCHEMISTRY IN NUTRITION

Biochemistry is a branch of science that studies the chemical processes and substances in living organisms. In nutrition, biochemistry can help us understand how the body utilizes nutrients from food and how different foods affect our metabolism and energy levels. This includes how different macronutrients (carbohydrates, proteins, and fats) and micronutrients (vitamins and minerals) are broken down and used by the body for energy and growth. Understanding nutrition's biochemistry also helps explain how certain nutritional deficiencies can lead to specific health problems and how certain dietary interventions may be used to prevent or treat these problems. Overall, awareness of biochemistry in nutrition is vital for promoting optimal health and preventing disease.

This knowledge can improve body composition, which refers to the ratio of muscle, fat, and other tissues. By better understanding the biochemistry of nutrition and how it relates to body composition, we can make more informed choices about what to eat and develop more effective weight loss and muscle-building strategies. For example, we know that certain nutrients, such as protein, can help increase muscle mass and reduce body fat. In contrast, other nutrients, such as simple sugars, can contribute to weight gain and negatively impact body composition. In this chapter, we'll investigate different factors that impact body composition a bit closer.

METABOLISM

Have you ever been curious about how some people seem to be able to eat everything without putting on weight? Some people, on the other hand, only need to look at the recipe to gain five pounds! This disparity can, in part, be explained by metabolism.

The easiest way to define metabolism is as the rate at which our bodies burn energy. Our genes determine our metabolism, and it is largely out of our control (*Does metabolism matter in weight loss?*, 2015). The operative word here is "largely," as there are some things we do that help or harm the metabolism, but we'll get to those in a moment. One way to explain metabolism is to compare it to a car engine or generator that is always running. Whether you are sitting still, doing the dishes, or sleeping, energy is being burned to keep the body's engine running. The fuel we add to the engine (in the form of food and drink) either gets burned quickly or stored for later use in the form of fat. How fast this engine runs essentially determines how many calories our bodies burn. Some people just have a fast metabolism, thanks to their genes, and burn more energy during rest and daily activities. A fast metabolism also means these individuals need to eat more to maintain their weight. On the other hand, when we have a slow metabolism, we'll need fewer calories on a daily basis to maintain our weight.

Understanding how the body metabolizes different nutrients, such as carbohydrates, proteins, and fats, can help us make better decisions about what to eat and how much to eat to maintain a healthy weight and body composition. There are ways we can help our metabolism, which includes understanding the following:

- **Energy balance:**

Understanding how energy balance affects body composition is important. Consuming the right amount of calories to match the energy expended can improve body composition. There are three ways we can safely change our energy balance. This is done mainly by changing our food intake, changing our exercise plans to maximize energy expenditure, and through increasing nonexercise activity (Dieter, n.d.). "Nonexercise activity" is just a different way of saying "move more throughout the day." Having a sedentary lifestyle reduces the amount of energy we burn and can negatively impact the metabolism. Finding creative ways to move more throughout the day can prove to be a fun and effective way to burn off extra energy.

- **Macronutrient balance:**

Body composition can be impacted by eating the proper combination of carbohydrates, proteins, and fats. For instance, meals high in protein may encourage muscle building while those low in carbohydrates may encourage fat reduction. Each of the macronutrients influence health in unique ways, but they all are sources of energy (Carreiro et al., 2016).

- **Micronutrient balance:**

Consuming the right balance of vitamins and minerals can improve metabolism, affecting body composition.

Our bodies can become deficient in micronutrients when we don't consume a healthy and balanced diet. It is believed that 10 million Americans are iron deficient, which is a serious condition because iron is a vital nutrient. (Miller, 2013). Our bodies struggle to deliver oxygen to the tissues that require it when we don't have enough iron, which can have an effect on all of the body's systems.

Zinc is yet another significant vitamin that affects metabolism. This nutrient supports insulin expression, plays a part in our immune system, and regulates how fats and sugars are metabolized (Ezzeldin, 2022). There are other micronutrients that also play a role in metabolism and the best way to get them is to eat a varied and balanced diet. In some cases, supplementation might be needed, but this should be done under the guidance of a trained medical professional.

- **Hormonal balance:**

Hormones such as insulin, cortisol, and thyroid hormones play a significant role in metabolism, and imbalances in these hormones can negatively affect body composition. Let's take a brief look at insulin. The hormone is secreted by the pancreas and responsible for the storage of glucose in the muscle, liver, and fat cells (Landes, 2022). The hormone is secreted in small amounts throughout the day, but greater quantities are released following meals. Depending on the body's needs, insulin will either transport glucose to our cells for energy or store it for later use. Insulin resistance is a condition when our cells become less responsive to the hormone and can lead to high blood sugar levels. As we know, high blood sugar levels can have devastating effects on the body.

- **Metabolic rate:**

Understanding the role of metabolism in the body can help optimize it to improve body composition. Our metabolism is a complicated process, and it may be divided into three basic components: basal metabolic rate (BMR), thermogenesis (the energy used to digest and absorb food), and the energy we expend during physical activity. The basal metabolic rate is believed to make up most of our daily energy use accounting for 50% to 80% of our daily energy use (*Metabolism*, 2012). Increasing lean muscle mass is one of the best and safest ways to increase our BMR.

- **Nutrient timing:**

Eating the right foods at the right time can help to opti-mize the body's metabolism and improve body composition. Given that metabolic disease and aging have a significant impact on our circadian rhythms, there is mounting evidence that the timing of meals is crucial for a healthy metabolism (Kessler & Pivovarova-Ramich, 2019).

- **Adequate hydration:**

Hydration is essential for metabolism and digestion and can help to improve body composition by keeping the body functioning optimally. Mild to severe dehydration can greatly slow down our metabolic rate, according to a number of studies (Puri, 2021). All the more reason to reach for a refreshing glass of water!

- **Genetics:**

Genetics plays a role in body composition, and understanding how genetics affects metabolism can help us to optimize our diet and exercise to improve body composition.

It is important to note that the most effective way to improve body composition is through a combination of diet, exercise, and lifestyle changes. Proper nutrition is essential for understanding how the body processes and utilizes the nutrients from food and how imbalances in nutrient intake can affect metabolism and body composition. This can help individuals make informed choices about their diet and eating habits, leading to optimal health and body composition.

ENERGY BALANCE

The balance between energy intake and expenditure is vital for maintaining a healthy body weight. Knowing how different types of foods and nutrients affect energy balance can help us make better choices about what to eat and how much to eat.

- **Caloric intake:** Understanding how many calories the body needs to maintain or change body composition is important. Consuming the right amount of calories to match the energy expended can improve body composition.
- **Macronutrient balance:** Consuming the right balance of carbohydrates, proteins, and fats can affect energy balance and body composition. For example, high-protein diets may promote muscle growth, while low-carb diets may promote fat loss.
- **Thermic effect of food:** Food's thermic effect is the energy required to digest, absorb, and metabolize food. Understanding how different types of foods affect the thermic effect of food

can help optimize energy balance and body composition. For example, protein can increase our metabolic rate by 15% to 30%, carbs by 5% to 10%, while fats only contribute a 3% increase (Dvorak, 2021). It is important to note that these increases are only temporary but can have a significant impact in the long run.

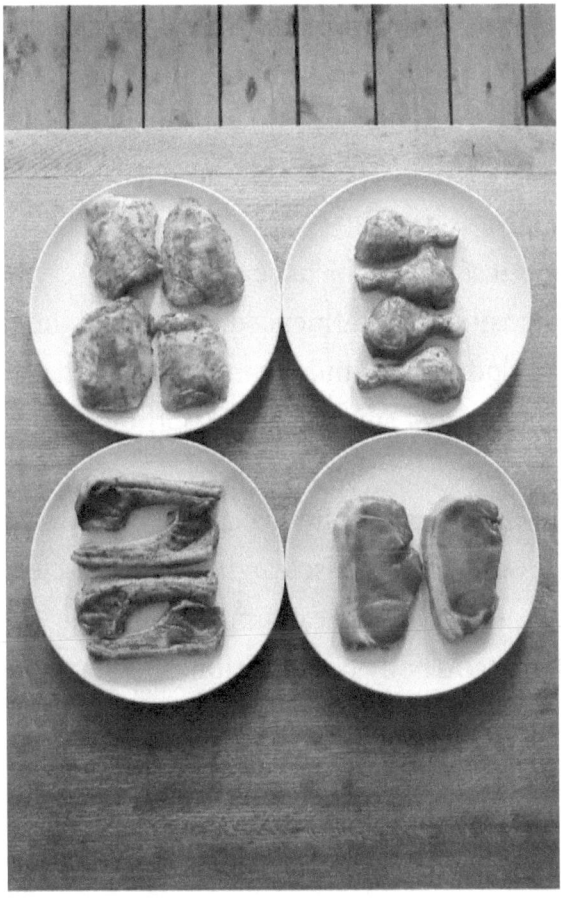

- **Metabolic rate:** It is possible to optimize metabolism to enhance energy balance and body composition by having a better understanding of its function in the body.
- **Nutrient timing:** The body's metabolism can be improved by eating the proper meals at the right times, which can also help with energy balance and body composition.
- **Adequate hydration:** Maintaining proper body function through hydration is important for digestion and metabolism and can assist to regulate energy levels and improve body composition.
- **Genetics:** Energy balance and body composition are influenced by genetics; hence, it is important to understand how genetics affect metabolism in order to optimize food and exercise for these goals.
- **Exercise:** Regular physical activity not only burns calories but also can increase muscle mass, which in turn can improve energy balance and body composition.

Again, it is important to note that the most effective way to improve body composition is through a combination of diet, exercise, and lifestyle changes. Consulting a professional such as a dietitian or a personal trainer would be beneficial to tailor a plan that suits your needs.

HORMONAL REGULATION

Hormones play a critical role in regulating metabolism and body weight. Understanding how different foods and nutrients affect hormone levels, such as insulin and leptin, can help us make better decisions about what to eat and how much to eat. When talking about hormones, the following factors need to be considered:

- **Hormone synthesis:** Biochemistry helps us understand how the body uses nutrients to synthesize hormones. For example, cholesterol is needed to produce steroid hormones such as testosterone, estrogen, and progesterone, which all play a role in body composition.
- **Metabolism of macronutrients:** Biochemistry can also help us understand how the body processes and utilizes carbohydrates, proteins, and fats can affect hormone regulation. For example, insulin is a hormone that regulates blood sugar levels and is affected by the consumption of carbohydrates, and an imbalance in insulin can lead to weight gain.

- **Metabolism of micronutrients:** Biochemistry helps us understand how the body processes and utilizes vitamins and minerals essential for hormone regulation. For example, vitamin D is involved in regulating parathyroid hormone, which helps regulate calcium metabolism, and a deficiency in vitamin D can lead to muscle loss.
- **Hormone signaling:** Biochemistry helps us understand how hormones interact with cells and tissues, which are necessary for hormone regulation. For example, insulin binds to cells and regulates glucose uptake, which is important for maintaining blood sugar levels and body composition.
- **Hormone breakdown:** Biochemistry helps us understand how the body breaks down hormones. For example, enzymes are involved in the breakdown of hormones, and nutrient deficiencies can lead to enzyme dysfunction and affect hormone regulation and body composition.
- **Hormone imbalance:** Lastly, biochemistry helps us understand how nutrient deficiencies or excesses can cause hormone imbalances, leading to weight gain or weight loss, and affect body composition.

Overall, a solid grasp of nutrition biochemistry is necessary to comprehend how the body absorbs nutrients from food and how nutrient imbalances can alter hormone control and body composition. This can assist people in making educated decisions regarding their diet and eating patterns, resulting in optimal health and body composition.

NUTRIENT TIMING

The timing of nutrient intake can have a significant impact on body composition. For example, consuming protein immediately after a workout can help promote muscle growth, while consuming carbohydrates before a workout can help improve performance. When considering the timing of nutrient intake, keep the following in mind:

- **The macronutrient composition:**

A meal's macronutrient balance can impact the body's insulin response, which in turn can impact fat storage, muscular growth, and recovery. For instance, taking carbs before and after exercise can enhance athletic performance and recovery by raising insulin sensitivity, while consuming a higher proportion of protein and fat can stimulate muscle protein synthesis and encourage muscle growth and repair.

- **The absorption rate:**

The body's insulin response and nutrient partitioning may be impacted by the rate at which macronutrients are absorbed. In contrast, consuming carbohydrates with a high GI can result in a rapid insulin response and nutrient partitioning towards fat storage. For instance, consuming carbohydrates with a low glycemic index (GI) can aid in promoting a slower insulin response and nutrient partitioning towards muscle growth and recovery.

- **The timing of nutrient consumption:**

The proper timing of macronutrient intake can influence fat loss, muscle growth and repair, and nutrient partitioning. For instance, eating carbohydrates before and after exercise can aid with athletic performance and recuperation, whereas eating protein right away after exercise can stimulate muscle growth and recovery.

- **The overall calorie intake:**

In addition to the macronutrient composition and timing of food consumption, the total amount of calories consumed also affects body composition. Eating too many calories might result in weight gain while eating too little calories can also adversely affect our bodies.

- **The overall macronutrient ratio:**

Consuming macronutrients in the right proportions can promote muscle development and recovery while reducing fat storage. A diet that is richer in protein and lower in carbohydrates, for instance, can encourage weight loss while helping to build and repair muscles.

By comprehending these factors and how they impact the body, people can employ nutrient timing to achieve their fitness objectives and enhance body composition. However, it is critical to remember that nutrient timing is insufficient on its own. It is important to take into account the overall calorie intake and nutritional makeup of a diet. Additionally, consulting a specialist is imperative because the timing and ratios of macronutrients might differ based on the individual and their goals and may not be appropriate for everyone. There is no one-size-fits-all solution, so it is important to cater to our unique needs.

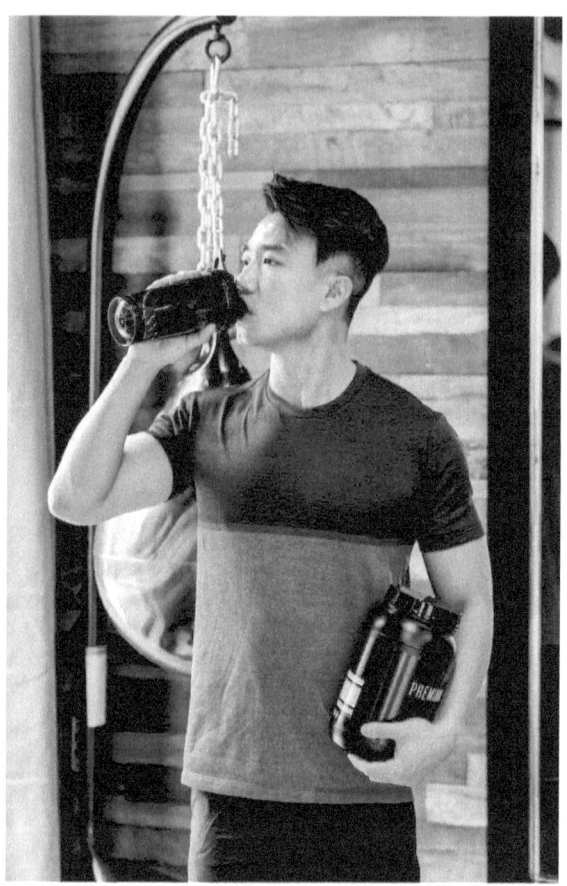

NUTRIENT DENSITY

Nutrient density refers to the number of nutrients in a food relative to its calorie content. Vegetables, whole grains, seafood, lean meats, peas, eggs, beans, nuts, and low-fat or fat-free milk products are all examples of nutrient-dense foods (*Nutrient-dense food*, 2011). Understanding nutrient density can help us make better choices about what to eat and ensure that we get the most nutritional bang for our calorie buck. When thinking about nutrient density, we need to consider the following factors:

- **Bioavailability:**

The amount of a nutrient that can be absorbed and utilized by the body is referred to as its bioavailability. Our food is categorized as being more nutrient-dense when its nutrients are more bioavailable. Macronutrients (carbs, fats and protein) have a high bioavailability and we tend to get all we need from a healthy diet. Other nutrients are a bit harder for our bodies to utilize.

Take the calcium in spinach as an example. Of all the leafy greens, spinach contains the most calcium, but our bodies can only make use of a tiny fraction of it (Khan Mirajkar, 2021). This happens because spinach contains anti-nutrients, which stop nutrients from being absorbed. If spinach was the only source of calcium we consumed, it could result in an insufficient calcium intake. The lesson here is not to shun spinach because it contains many beneficial elements but to eat a range of foods so that our bodies may get the nutrients they need.

- **Micronutrient density:**

The micronutrient density of a food refers to the number of essential vitamins and minerals it contains. Foods that are high in micronutrients are considered more nutrient-dense. Some of the best food sources for micronutrients include small fish, organ meats (such as liver), dark leafy greens, crustaceans, bivalves, beef, eggs, milk, mutton, lamb, canned fish with bones, cheese and goat milk (Beal & Ortenzi, 2022).

- **Fiber content:**

Fiber is an important nutrient that helps promote satiety and gut health. Foods that are high in fiber are considered more nutrient-dense. Fiber is crucial for a healthy digestive system, as it feeds friendly gut bacteria (Gunnars, 2018). Additionally, fiber can aid in weight loss, blood sugar control, and constipation relief. High-fiber foods include avocado, chia seeds, raspberries, bananas, artichoke, carrots, beets, lentils, kidney beans, split peas, chickpeas, oats, almonds, sweet potatoes and pears.

- **Antioxidant content:**

The body is protected by antioxidants against oxidative damage and inflammation. Antioxidant-rich foods are also considered to be higher in nutrients. There are plenty of foods that are high in antioxidants. As a general rule, foods that are rich in vibrant hues, such as orange, yellow, blue, and red, tend to be higher in antioxidants. With so many colorful food options, you'll never get bored or run out of delectable meal ideas! Blueberries, red kidney beans, cranberries, artichokes, black plums, prunes, and dark leafy greens are only a small handful of the options available (Reilly, n.d.).

- **Macronutrient ratio:**

The macronutrient ratio of a food can affect its nutrient density. For example, a food high in protein and low in carbohydrates can be considered more nutrient-dense than one high in carbohydrates and low in protein.

- **Processing level:**

Processed foods tend to have lower nutrient density than whole foods. Whole foods are generally considered more nutrient-dense than their processed counterparts. So, try to incorporate more whole foods into your diets and steer clear from processed foods as much as possible.

It's important to note that nutrient density is different from calorie density. Nutrient-dense foods provide a lot of essential nutrients for the number of calories they contain, while calorie-dense foods are high in calories but low in essential nutrients.

FOOD QUALITY

The quality of the foods we eat can significantly impact our health and body composition. Understanding the different types of nutrients in food and their bioavailability can help us make better choices about what to eat. When we talk about the "quality" of food, it is important to consider the following:

- **Nutrient density:** Food quality is closely related to nutrient density, which refers to the amount of essential vitamins, minerals, and other nutrients a food contains per calorie. Nutrient-dense foods are considered higher quality than those low in essential nutrients.
- **Processing level:** Processing can deplete the nutrient density of foods and also could add unwanted additives, preservatives, and artificial

ingredients. Whole foods are considered to be of higher quality than their processed counterparts.

- **Organic vs. conventional:** Organic foods are grown without synthetic pesticides and fertilizers and are considered higher quality than conventional foods. Organic produce can be expensive, so it is encouraged to grow your own whenever possible.

- **Antioxidant content:** Antioxidants protect the body against oxidative stress and inflammation. Foods that are high in antioxidants are considered to be of higher quality than those that are low in antioxidants.

- **Micronutrient density:** The micronutrient density of a food refers to the amount of essential vitamins and minerals it contains. Foods that are high in micronutrients are considered to be of higher quality than those that are low in micronutrients.

- **Food origin and freshness:** Foods grown locally and consumed when fresh are considered higher quality than those grown far away and are not consumed when they are fresh.

It's important to remember that the definition of "food quality" can vary depending on the context. Personal preferences and dietary restrictions can influence the definition as well.

SUPPLEMENTATION

To meet their dietary objectives, some individuals may think about taking dietary supplements. It's critical to comprehend how various supplements interact with the body, as well as any potential adverse effects and suggested dosages. For this reason, we need to consider the following before taking any supplements:

- **Nutrient deficiencies:** Supplementation can be used to correct deficiencies that may prevent optimal body composition. For example, supplementing with iron can help improve athletic performance in individuals with iron-deficiency anemia.
- **Absorption:** The bioavailability and absorption of the nutrient in supplement form can affect its effectiveness. For example, some forms of a nutrient may be more bioavailable and absorbable than others, affecting its effectiveness in promoting body composition goals.

- **Dosage:** The dosage of a nutrient in supplement form can affect its effectiveness. Too little of a nutrient may not be practical, while too much can be harmful. It is important to consult with a healthcare professional before starting any supplement regimen.
- **Interactions:** Some supplements may interact with medications or other supplements, affecting their effectiveness or safety. This is why speaking to a healthcare professional beforehand is so important.
- **Quality:** The quality of the supplement can affect its effectiveness. It's important to choose supplements manufactured by reputable companies and verified by third-party organizations like USP and NSF.
- **Timing:** The timing of nutrient supplementation can also affect its effectiveness. For example, consuming a protein supplement immediately after exercise can help support muscle recovery and growth, while consuming it at other times may not be as effective.

It's crucial to remember that supplements should be taken in addition to an exercise regimen and are not intended as a replacement for a healthy diet. Before beginning any supplement program, it is vital to speak with a healthcare expert because, depending on an individual's health situation, some supplements may not be suitable.

Understanding the biochemistry of nutrition can help us make better judgments about what to eat and create more efficient weight reduction and muscle-building techniques. By better understanding how the body metabolizes different nutrients, how energy balance is affected by food choices, and how hormones regulate metabolism and body weight, we can make better choices about what to eat and how much to eat. Additionally, by paying attention to nutrient timing, nutrient density, food quality, and supplementation, we can support our body in reaching its optimal state. Overall, understanding the biochemistry of nutrition can help us achieve our goals related to weight loss and body composition and improve our overall health.

FOOD DIARY-BASED ACTION

In this activity we will build on what we've learned in the previous chapters by adding one last element: A section to document our activity. As in the previous chapters, we'll rate our hunger, inspect our emotions and carefully document the meals we've eaten.

Meal	How Hungry I Felt (scored from 1–10)	Food Consumed	Amount Consumed	How Satiated I Felt (scored from 1–10)	Did I Eat My Emotions? How did I feel afterwards?
Breakfast	3	Muesli and coffee.	One serving of muesli and a cup of coffee with two teaspoons of sugar and milk.	8	I ate because I was hungry.
Lunch	5	Spicy taco and Coke.	One taco (prepared by a street vendor) and a bottle of diet Coke.	9	I didn't pack a lunch, so I grabbed something tasty from the food vendor nearby. I ate because I was
Dinner	5	Roast chicken and vegetables with some juice.	Had a chicken thigh with roast vegetables (prepared at home) and cranberry juice.	9	Today was a great day! I didn't eat my emotions or overeat. I only ate when I was hungry.

How Do I Feel About My Body Today? Why?			What Exercise Did I Do Today? How Did I Feel Afterwards?		
Today I feel comfortable in my skin. I like what I see in the mirror!			*I went for a three-mile walk. It took me nearly two hours and I struggled. It was worth it, though, because I felt great afterwards!*		
Breakfast					
Lunch					
Dinner					
How Do I Feel About My Body Today? Why?			**What Exercise Did I Do Today? How Did I Feel Afterwards?**		

5

IT'S ABOUT YOUR BASELINE DIETARY NUTRITION

The bare minimum of nutrients that a person requires to stay healthy and avoid nutrient deficits is referred to as baseline nutrition. Carbohydrates, proteins, lipids, vitamins, and minerals are some of these nutrients. The Recommended Dietary Allowance (RDA) and the Adequate Intake (AI) provide the recommended daily intake of essential nutrients for different age groups and genders. However, it's important to note that these guidelines are just that, a guideline and may not be appropriate for everyone. Individual needs can vary based on factors such as age, sex, activity level, and health status. To establish personal baseline nutrition, it's recommended to consult with a dietitian or a nutritionist who can assess your dietary habits, medical history, and any other relevant information to determine your specific nutrient needs.

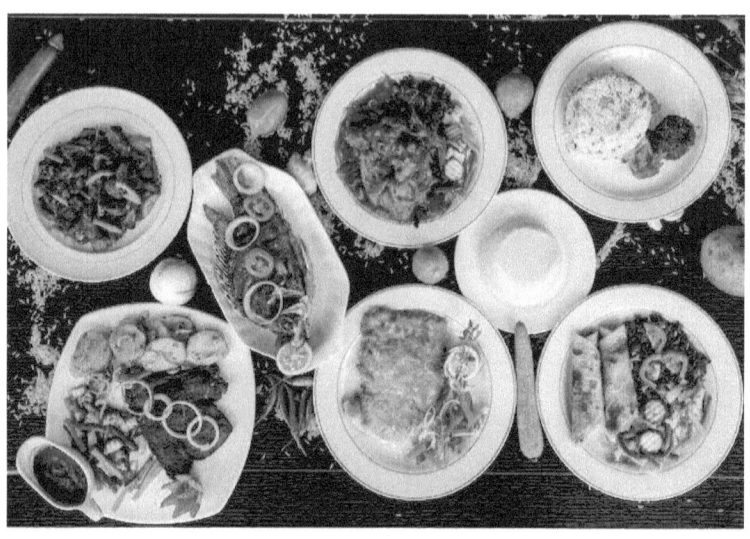

It's also critical to keep in mind that having a healthy diet means getting the recommended amount of nutrients as well as a balance of meals that provide you both the energy and nutrition you need. A balanced diet must contain a range of foods from all the food groups, including lean proteins, whole grains, fruits, vegetables, and healthy fats. You'll have more energy, be in a better mood, and have a more youthful appearance with a diet that is adapted to your needs. With that being said, let's get better acquainted with the concept of baseline nutrition.

THE IMPORTANCE OF KNOWING YOUR BASELINE NUTRITION

For your future health objectives to be successful, establishing your baseline is essential. Many health and wellness goals start with radical food and exercise changes, but your healthcare practitioner can help you assess whether these changes are safe (or even necessary). You might be saying to yourself, "I've never needed to go to a hospital, and I don't take any medications. Why should I start going to a doctor now?" This is a valid and important question. We need to remember that preventative care and appropriate treatment for present illnesses serve as the two pillars that sustain good health. Preventative care is frequently neglected, which increases the risk of subsequent health issues. Because the body's requirements fluctuate over time, part of preventative care includes becoming familiar with our baseline nutrition. The factors to consider when establishing our baseline nutrition include the following:

- **Age:** Nutritional needs vary by age, with different recommendations for infants, children, teenagers, adults, and seniors.
- **Gender:** Men and women have different nutritional needs and varying calorie and nutrient recommendations.
- **Pregnancy and breastfeeding:** Women who are pregnant or breastfeeding have increased nutritional needs.
- **Activity level:** Physical activity can affect your nutritional needs, so it's important to consider this when evaluating your baseline dietary nutrition.
- **Medical conditions:** If you have any medical conditions, such as diabetes, it's important to consult with a healthcare professional to determine the dietary recommendations that are specific to you.
- **Medications:** Certain medications can affect nutrient absorption or increase the need for certain nutrients, so it's important to be aware of your medications and how they may affect your nutritional needs.
- **Personal preferences and cultural food habits:** Some people may have specific dietary restrictions, allergies, or food preferences that affect their nutritional needs, and it's important

to consider these when determining your baseline nutrition.

- **Body composition:** Your body composition (BMI, body fat, muscle mass) can affect your nutritional needs, so it's important to consider this when determining your baseline nutrition.

You must continue as directed by your healthcare professional after your baseline has been determined. People with complicated medical issues could require numerous follow-ups. It's critical to follow up to make sure we're taking care of our bodies's evolving demands so we can maintain optimal health.

ONE SIZE DOES NOT FIT ALL

A diet and exercise routine are often the first steps toward achieving a health objective. Many people often turn to the internet to download a generic wellness plan to help them on this journey. There is just one problem: A general wellness plan with diet and exercise advice does not take your particular needs into consideration. In order to reach our health objectives as effectively as possible, it is necessary for us to establish our baseline. The dietary and exercise modifications you need to make should be decided with the aid of your primary care physician. Keep in mind that mental and emotional health are also important steps on the path to wellness. Get the necessary treatment if depression, anxiety, or other problems are present. When assessing your individual needs, the following factors need to be taken into account:

- **Prevention of nutrient deficiencies:** By understanding your baseline nutrition, you can ensure that you get the minimum essential nutrients needed to maintain good health and prevent nutrient deficiencies.
- **Achieving optimal health:** A balanced diet that includes a variety of foods from all food groups can help you achieve optimal health and prevent chronic diseases.
- **Achieving your health goals:** Knowing your baseline nutrition can help you achieve specific health goals, such as losing weight, building muscle, or managing a medical condition.
- **Making informed food choices:** Understanding your baseline nutrition can help you make informed food choices, such as selecting foods that provide the necessary nutrients and energy and avoiding foods that may trigger allergic reactions or other health issues.

- **Monitoring your progress:** Knowing your baseline nutrition can help you track your progress and adjust your diet.
- **Being aware of any food allergies, sensitivities, or restrictions:** By knowing your baseline nutrition, you can identify any food allergies, sensitivities, or restrictions and adjust your diet accordingly. Food allergies can sneak up on us without warning, as it did with me. Honeydew melon used to be one of my favorite fruits, but one day after thoroughly enjoying some of the fruit I found myself gasping for air. My throat and eyes were swollen shut and I had to be rushed to the emergency room. Turns out I had a severe allergy to honeydew melon! This dangerous situation could have been prevented had I gone for the allergy tests my doctor recommended a long time ago. There is no known cure for food allergies, so individuals with allergies are strongly advised to listen to their healthcare provider's instructions. Please don't make the same mistake I did. Allergies can be life-threatening.
- **Being aware of any nutrient deficiencies:** By knowing your baseline nutrition, you can identify any nutrient deficiencies and take steps

to correct them, such as by taking supplements or making dietary adjustments.

Bear in mind that your body and your circumstances are unique. It would, therefore, be unreasonable to expect favorable results from generic wellness plans. By establishing your baseline, it is possible to tailor your nutritional intake to promote optimal health. The results may pleasantly surprise you!

IMPROVE YOUR BASELINE NUTRITION

Now that we have a good idea of what baseline nutrition is, there are steps we can take to improve it. These steps are simple and form a natural part of a healthy lifestyle. The steps we can take to improve our overall health and nutritional status include:

- **Keep a food diary:**

Writing down all of what you eat and drink for a week, including the time of day, portion size, and other relevant information. This will give you a clear picture of your current dietary habits. The food-diary based action at the end of each chapter is designed to help you focus on key areas that impact food choices and body composition the most.

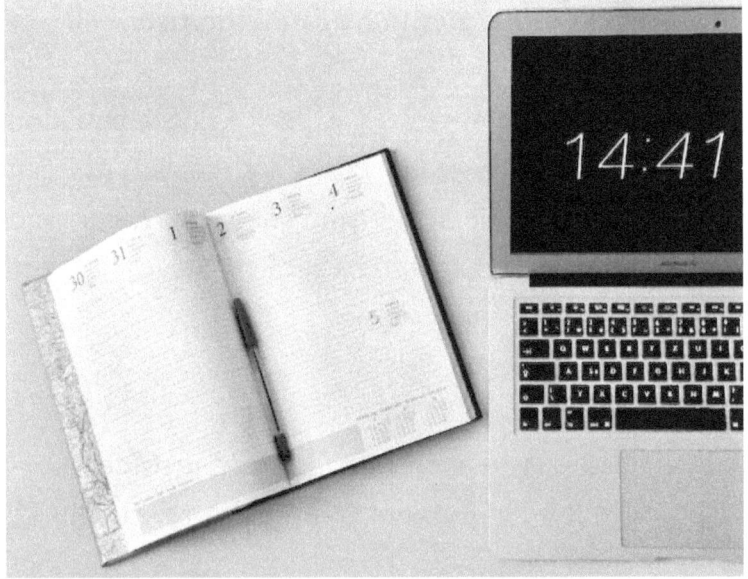

- **Review your food diary:**

Look for patterns and identify areas where you may lack essential nutrients, such as fruits, vegetables, lean protein, or whole grains. Reviewing the food diary can also reveal if we've been engaging in emotional eating or if we've been neglecting exercise plans. Try to review your food diary once a week. This will give you a good (and honest) depiction of how your week went. If the results are not what you expected, don't be too hard on yourself. Remember, you are on a journey of personal growth. Meaningful change does not happen overnight, but we can build on small gains to attain our goals.

- **Consult with a dietitian or nutritionist:**

They can provide you with a personalized nutrition plan based on your health needs and goals. They can also help you understand your nutrient needs and provide guidance on how to meet them.

- **Get a blood test:**

A blood test can be very revealing and provide information about your nutrient levels, such as vitamin D, Iron, vitamin B12, and other micronutrients. Think of these blood tests as a window to the inner workings of your body. We need them to fine-tune our nutritional approach so that we can enjoy optimal health in the long run. Also, bloodwork is handy to spot and curb potential health problems early on, for example the development of diabetes or cholesterol that can lead to cardiac problems. Don't worry, you won't need to get a blood test every month (unless your doctor advises otherwise). At the very minimum we need to get bloodwork done once a year (Griffin, 2022).

- **Assess your physical activity:**

Your physical activity level can affect your nutritional needs, so it's important to consider this when evaluating your baseline dietary nutrition. Not all forms of exercise are suitable for everyone, for example individuals with chronic pain, knee injuries, or an injured back won't be able to perform certain exercises. It is recommended to speak to your healthcare provider before starting a fitness plan as it is possible that some exercises need to be modified or removed for safety reasons.

- **Take into account any medical conditions:**

If you have any medical conditions, such as diabetes or cardiac issues, it is vital to note that the nutritional needs can and do vary.

Factors such as age, sex, activity level, and health status all impact our baseline nutritional needs. Therefore, it's essential to consult with a healthcare professional to determine the appropriate baseline for you.

FOOD DIARY-BASED ACTION

Having a good understanding of our baseline nutritional needs can significantly impact the results we hope to achieve. In this chapter's food-diary activity we won't be introducing any new sections to fill in. Instead, reflect on the following questions as you complete your food diary for the day:

- **When was the last time I had a proper check-up?** If you can't remember or if it was more than a year ago, then perhaps it's time to make an appointment.
- **When was the last time I had bloodwork done?** Again, if you can't remember or if this happened more than a year ago, it is advised to get this done as well.
- **How can I improve my daily nutrition?** If you are unsure how to go about this, it is advised to speak to a dietician.

Eating nutrient-dense meals (as described in the previous chapter), limiting our consumption of processed foods, and making sure we drink enough water are some easy steps we can take to improve our daily nutrition.

Meal	How Hungry I Felt (scored from 1–10)	Food Consumed	Amount Consumed	How Satiated I Felt (scored from 1–10)	Did I Eat My Emotions? How did I feel afterwards?
Breakfast	4	Whole grain muffin and coffee.	One whole grain muffin (purchased at a convenience store) and a coffee with sugar and milk.	6	Had a very light breakfast because I was late for work. Ate because I was hungry.
Lunch	1	Steak, vegetables, and a chocolate milkshake.	One sirloin steak, spinach, beets, and a chocolate milkshake (prepared by restaurant).	9	I was ravenous! I tried to order filling, healthy food. The milkshake was just a treat.
Dinner	5	Toasted cheese sandwiches and juice.	Two toasted cheese sandwiches on whole grain bread (prepared at home) and a glass of orange juice.	8	Today was a great day! I didn't overeat or eat my emotions.

How Do I Feel About My Body Today? Why?			What Exercise Did I Do Today? How Did I Feel Afterwards?		
I feel good. A little bit tired from having a busy day, but overall I feel good about myself.			*I did 30 minutes of yoga. Felt so relaxed afterwards!*		
Breakfast					
Lunch					
Dinner					
How Do I Feel About My Body Today? Why?			**What Exercise Did I Do Today? How Did I Feel Afterwards?**		

SHARE THE SEVEN FACTORS THAT STOP OTHERS FROM ACHIEVING THEIR DREAM BODY

"If we could give every individual the right amount of nourishment and exercise, not too little and not too much, we would have the safest way to health."

— HIPPOCRATES

The media often sells "one-size-fits-all" solutions for health and weight loss, yet as you will have discovered by now, acing your nutritional regime is anything but a "standard journey."

There are defined, proven reasons why you make specific food choices. Your social environment, biology, and attitudes and beliefs all influence the extent to which you prioritize health.

For instance, if your social life is centered around dining out at gourmet restaurants with friends, then you may be more likely to indulge in rich, calorific meals.

If you are an active athlete, meanwhile, then you may be a whiz on aspects such as macronutrients and micronutrients and the way they can shape your body and bring you closer to your goals.

For most people, finding the right nutritional plan is a journey of discovery. By knowing how the seven factors revealed in this book influence your food choices, you can design a personalized nutritional plan that takes your lifestyle, values, and goals into account.

Becoming knowledgeable about the type of fuel that can power your body to better physical and mental health puts you in a unique position to help those who are just starting out on their journey. Many people make food choices based on impulse or psychological factors. They may be unaware of the powerful influence that factors such as societal pressure, nutrient timing, or their baseline nutrition have over them.

This is where your valuable help can turn their life around.

By letting them know the secrets of why they are drawn to certain foods, you can inspire them to take a more proactive role in their nutritional journey.

By leaving a review of this book on the bookseller's website where you purchased it, you can help people identify negative eating habits, create a bespoke nutritional plan, and achieve their health or weight loss goals.

Simply by sharing how this book has helped you and what information you found here, you'll help other readers find the guidance they seek.

Nutrition is power, and you can ensure that more people harness it to live more purposefully, mindfully, and energetically. Thank you for joining me on my mission to help people live longer and better.

6

GOING BACK TO THE BASICS OF NUTRITION

Healthy nutrition is the foundation of good health; there's no denying that. The challenge in today's fast-paced world is to eat a balanced diet to provide our bodies with all the nutrients they need to remain healthy. In this context, "Going Back to the Basics of Nutrition" is a method or approach to nutrition that emphasizes the importance of understanding the fundamentals of good nutrition and applying them to your daily life. Nutrient-dense foods include protein, omega-3 fatty acids, iron, vitamin D, magnesium, copper, selenium, zinc, and other nutrients. Balanced meals include adequate protein, calcium, and healthy carbohydrates in the right proportions. By going back to the basics of nutrition, we can make informed decisions about what we eat and develop long-term healthy eating habits that will support our overall well-being.

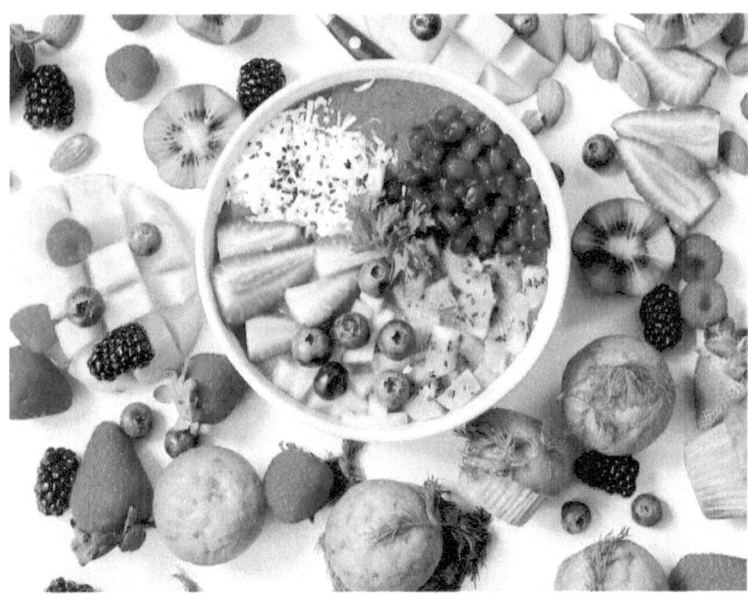

Fruits, vegetables, whole grains, lean meats, and healthy fats are some foods emphasized in this chapter. Good health can be maintained with these foods's essential vitamins, minerals, and other essential nutrients. Bear in mind that the basics of nutrition do not allow for the consumption of added sugars, saturated fats, or processed foods. The goal is to keep our foods wholesome and unprocessed. Overeating on foods rich in sugars and saturated fats contributes significantly to weight gain and chronic disease (*Obesity*, 2019). For this reason, it is strongly recommended to steer clear of processed foods, as they are typically filled with unhealthy fats and sugars. Think of these foods as "empty energy sources," i.e., they are low in essential nutrients but high in calories.

Staying within your daily calories and paying attention to portion sizes are some things to keep in mind. This can help maintain a healthy weight and prevent overeating. Additionally, staying hydrated is an essential part of a balanced diet. Our bodies need good old H_2O to function properly. National health organizations such as the FDA, USDA, and the WHO have set guidelines for food and drink intake. These guidelines give us the broad idea of the nutrients that the average, healthy individual needs and is a good starting point. A registered dietitian or healthcare professional can help you develop a personalized nutrition plan that works for you. Rather than following a fad diet or restrictive eating plan, you should adopt a long-term, sustainable approach to healthy eating. By following these guidelines, you can go back to the basics of nutrition and develop a healthy relationship with food that will support your overall well-being. With that being said, let's get better acquainted with the important nutrients our bodies need.

FUNCTIONS OF CARBOHYDRATES

Carbs have a rightful place in a healthy diet, despite what proponents of "low carb" and "zero carb" eating plans might say. That's because carbohydrates (along with proteins and fats) provide the body with energy. So what exactly are carbohydrates, and why did they get such a bad rap? We need to understand that carbs are a macronutrient that is present in many foods. Most carbs can be found in plant-based foods. These are the "good carbs." The "bad carbs" typically originate from added sugars that food manufacturers love to add to processed foods. All told, there are three main sources of carbohydrates:

- **Fiber:** This is classified as a complex carbohydrate and occurs naturally in fruit, whole grains, and vegetables. Our bodies can't digest fiber, but we need it to maintain a healthy digestive tract. When our diets are lacking in fiber we may experience problems like constipation. We'll discuss fiber in more detail later in the chapter.
- **Sugar:** This is the simplest form of carbs. It occurs naturally in certain foods like fruit, milk, and vegetables. The types of sugar we typically encounter are fructose (fruit sugar), sucrose

(table sugar), and lactose (milk sugar). Sugars are an energy source that is easily accessible to our bodies.

- **Starch:** This is classified as a complex carbohydrate. This is just another way of saying there's a lot of sugar molecules bonded together to create a starch molecule. Starch can naturally be found in grains, vegetables, peas and cooked dry beans. Our bodies need to work a bit harder to make use of starches, but it remains a relatively easily accessible energy source.

Common sources of carbs in a healthy diet include nuts, milk, vegetables, fruits, seeds, and grains. When wandering down the health food aisle of your grocery store, you might come across descriptions such as "low carb" or "net carbs" on food labels. Keep in mind that these descriptions do not have a standard meaning as the Food and Drug Administration does not use these terms (*Carbohydrates: how carbs fit into a healthy diet,* 2022). There are descriptions we often find on food items marketed towards a low-carb or zero-carb eating plan. The problem here is that these eating plans can misrepresent the importance of carbs, understating their importance to the body. The primary function of carbs is to produce hormones and keep the body strong. Unless your healthcare provider advises you otherwise, don't cut all carbs out of your life. Rather, try to enjoy them in moderation.

The Good of Carbohydrates

Now that we have a better idea of what carbohydrates are, let's take a closer look at the reasons why we should include them in our diet.

- **Provides energy:** Source of energy for the body. They are broken down into glucose, the primary energy source for the brain and muscles.
- **Maintains blood sugar levels:** Carbs help to regulate blood sugar levels by providing a steady source of glucose to the body.
- **Supports physical activity:** Carbohydrates are an essential fuel source for physical activity, particularly for endurance exercise.
- **Supports brain function:** Carbs are a vital energy source for the brain, without them the brain will have a hard time to function optimally.
- **Supports gut health:** Carbohydrates play a role in maintaining gut health by providing a source of fuel for beneficial gut bacteria.

- **Supports heart health:** High-fiber carbohydrates, such as whole grains, fruits, and vegetables, are associated with a reduced risk of heart disease.
- **Encourages satiety:** Carbohydrates also regulate appetite by providing a feeling of fullness and satisfaction after eating. This is why a high-fiber meal will leave us feeling fuller for longer.

The Bad of Carbohydrates

While carbohydrates are an essential macronutrient that provides energy for the body and supports overall health, there are also some potential downsides to consuming too many carbohydrates. Some of the main drawbacks of carbohydrates include:

- **Weight gain:** Consuming too many carbohydrates, particularly those high in added sugar or refined grains, can contribute to weight gain.
- **Blood sugar fluctuations:** Consuming high amounts of refined carbohydrates can cause spikes in blood sugar levels and contribute to insulin resistance, leading to type 2 diabetes.

- **Increased risk of chronic diseases:**
  Consuming too many refined carbohydrates
  may increase the risk of chronic diseases like
  heart disease, stroke, and certain cancers.
- **Nutrient deficiencies:** Consuming too many
  refined carbohydrates can displace nutrient-
  dense foods in the diet, leading to deficiencies
  in essential vitamins and minerals.
- **Dependence on carbohydrates for energy:**
  Some people may depend on carbohydrates to
  provide energy, decreasing physical and mental
  performance.

It's important to note that not all carbohydrates are
created equal, and it's important to choose nutrient-
dense carbohydrates such as fruits, vegetables, whole
grains, and legumes rather than those high in added
sugar or refined grains.

FUNCTIONS OF PROTEINS

Proteins are large, complex molecules that perform a
variety of functions in the body. They do most of the
heavy lifting in cells and are needed for the structure,
regulation, and function of organs and bodily tissues
(*What are proteins and what do they do?*, 2021). Proteins
are built from lengthy chains of smaller building blocks

called amino acids. There are a total of 20 different kinds of amino acids, which, when combined, produce various proteins. The easiest way to categorize proteins is to look at the functions they perform in the body. When looking at the functions, we'll find that proteins include:

- **Antibodies and enzymes:** Antibodies help to protect the body from viruses and bacteria, whilst enzymes play a key role in chemical reactions in cells.
- **Messengers:** These proteins, which include some hormones, play a role in the normal and healthy functioning of cells, tissues and organs.
- **Structural components:** Proteins provide structure and lend support to cells. They are also the building blocks of muscle, so without proteins we won't be able to move.
- **Transportation and storage:** The proteins involved in these functions see to it that atoms and other small molecules are transported throughout the body.

The Good of Proteins

Proteins are essential building blocks to maintain optimal health. Without them, our bodies will be hard-pressed to function normally. Now that we are better acquainted with this vital nutrient, let's take a closer look at all the good it does in our bodies.

- **Builds and repairs bodily tissues:** Proteins are essential for the growth, repair, and maintenance of body tissues, such as muscles, bones, skin, and hair.
- **Plays a role in metabolism:** Proteins act as enzymes, catalyzing metabolic reactions and hormones and regulating various bodily functions.
- **Transporting and storing molecules:** Proteins act as carriers, transport, and storage molecules, such as hemoglobin, which carries oxygen in the blood, and ferritin, which stores iron.
- **Immune system support:** Proteins, such as antibodies, play a crucial role in the immune system, which protects the body from harmful pathogens.
- **Fluid balance:** Proteins help maintain fluid balance in the body, such as albumin, which helps keep fluid in the blood vessels.
- **Encourages satiety:** Proteins are known to make you feel full and satisfied for a longer

time, which can be helpful for weight
management.

- **Maintaining healthy skin, hair, and nails:**
  Proteins are the building blocks of skin, hair,
  and nails and are essential for maintenance and
  repair.

The Bad of Proteins

Proteins are key macronutrients required for numerous
physiological activities, but consuming too much can
lead to potential negative effects. Before you start
downing protein smoothies like they're going out of
style, consider some of the negative effects of
consuming too much protein. These drawbacks include:

- **Kidney damage:** Consuming excessive
  amounts of protein, particularly animal protein,
  can strain the kidneys, leading to damage over
  time, especially in people with pre-existing
  kidney problems.
- **Dehydration:** A high-protein diet can lead to
  dehydration as the body needs more water to
  metabolize protein than carbohydrates or fats.
- **Increased risk of cancer:** Some studies have
  suggested that a diet high in animal protein

may increase the risk of certain types of cancer, such as colon and breast cancer (*Red Meat and Colon Cancer*, 2008).

- **Decrease in bone density:** A high-protein diet can increase acidity in the body, which can cause the bones to release calcium, reducing bone density.
- **Displace nutrient-dense foods:** Consuming too much protein can displace nutrient-dense foods in the diet, leading to deficiencies in essential vitamins and minerals.

It's vital to choose protein sources that are high in nutrients, such as lean meats, fish, eggs, beans, and legumes. Stick to the daily protein requirements recommended by national health organizations, and try to avoid foods high in saturated fats. With the help of a registered dietitian or another healthcare professional, you can design a personalized nutrition plan that is specific to your needs.

FUNCTIONS OF FATS

The macronutrient we love to hate! Fats, also known as lipids, are one of the three macronutrients (along with carbohydrates and proteins) that provide energy for the body. A balanced diet must include a small quantity of healthy fats. That's because dietary fats are a source of essential fatty acids, which the body cannot produce on its own. Furthermore, fat aids the absorption of certain vitamins. Any dietary fat that is not utilized by your body's cells or converted into energy is transformed into body fat, but the same goes for unused proteins and carbs (*Fat: The Facts*, 2022).

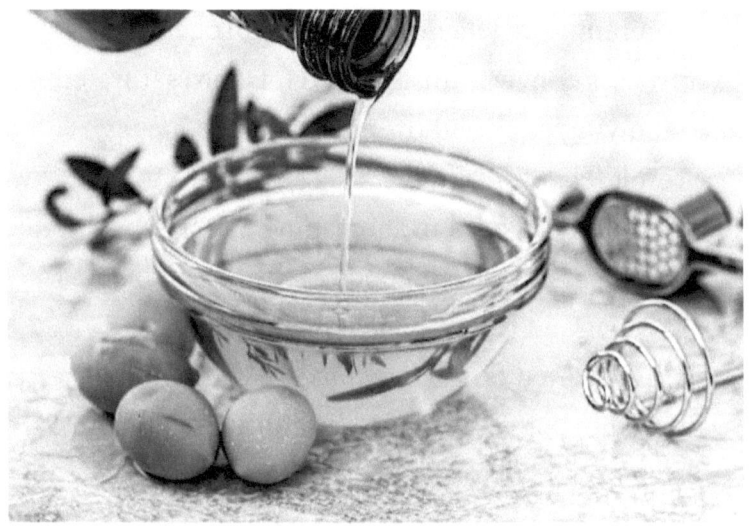

The main types of fat that we find in food include:

- **Saturated fats:** These fats are commonly found in sweet and savory foods. This fat is mostly derived from fatty cuts of meat, butter, ghee, lard, dairy products, palm oil, and coconut oils.

- **Trans fats:** These fats occur at low levels naturally in some foods, such as meat and dairy. Hydrogenated vegetable oils, on the other hand, are a major source of trans fats. Food items that contain hydrogenated or partly hydrogenated oil must declare the ingredient on the label, as too much trans fats can have a negative impact on our health. Hydrogenated fat is created by combining vegetable oils with hydrogen. This process converts unsaturated fats into saturated fat giving us a solid or semi-solid product as a result (*Fat hydrogenation*, 2021). Trans fats are the main fats used in shortening and most commercially baked goods as they tend to be cheaper and have a longer shelf-life.
- **Unsaturated fats:** These fats are commonly found in plants and fish. Unsaturated fats can be monounsaturated (olive oil, avocados, almonds, peanuts and Brazil nuts) or polyunsaturated (omega-3 and omega-6). Fatty fish, such as mackerel and salmon, are excellent sources of omega-3. These fats are generally considered to be heart-friendly and can improve cholesterol levels.

The Good of Fats

Despite being a necessary ingredient in a nutritious and well-balanced diet, fat has such a terrible reputation. Remember that fat is a food that contains a lot of energy, therefore a little bit goes a long way. Fat plays in essential role in our bodies by:

- **Providing energy:** Fats are an important source of energy for the body and are essential for maintaining physical and mental function.
- **Creating insulation and regulating temperature:** Fats insulate and protect the body by helping to maintain body temperature. We can think of fat as the body's shock absorber. This is why certain body parts and vital organs (like the kidneys) have a protective layer of fat. Without this protective layer these body parts are far more susceptible to injury and damage.
- **Supporting cell growth and development:** Fats are a cell membrane component essential for proper cell growth and development.
- **Aiding in the absorption of fat-soluble vitamins:** Some vitamins are water-soluble, like vitamin C. Others are fat-soluble. So, fat

plays an important role in the absorption of vitamins A, D, E, and K.

- **Supporting heart health:** Fats play a role in supporting heart health. Unsaturated fats, such as monounsaturated and polyunsaturated fats, can help lower harmful cholesterol levels, inflammation, and heart disease risk.
- **Encouraging satiety:** Fats can make you feel full and satisfied for a longer time, which can be helpful for weight management.

The Bad of Fats

While fat is an essential macronutrient that provides energy for the body and plays important roles in many physiological processes. There are also some potential downsides to consuming too much fat. Some of the main cons of fats include:

- **Weight gain:** Consuming too many fats, particularly saturated and trans fats, can contribute to weight gain and obesity.
- **Increased risk of chronic diseases:** Too much saturated and trans fats may increase the risk of chronic diseases such as heart disease, stroke, and certain cancers.

- **Blood lipid abnormalities:** Consuming too much saturated and trans fats can increase LDL (bad) cholesterol levels in the blood, leading to an increased risk of heart disease.
- **Nutrient deficiencies:** Consuming too many fats can displace nutrient-dense foods in the diet, leading to deficiencies in essential vitamins and minerals.
- **Inadequate essential fatty acids intake:** Not consuming enough foods such as nuts, seeds, and fatty fish can lead to deficiencies and health problems.

Instead of trans and saturated fats, choose monounsaturated and polyunsaturated fats. Foods like butter, cheese, nuts, seeds, avocados, and fatty seafood are good sources of healthy fats. Additionally, it's crucial to adhere to national health organization's recommendations for daily fat intake and work with a registered dietitian or other healthcare professional to create a specialized dietary plan. Fats are healthy and necessary for optimal health, but only when consumed in moderation.

FUNCTIONS OF DIETARY FIBER

As discussed earlier, dietary fiber is a carbohydrate found in plant-based foods that is not digested by the body. So why do we need fiber if the body can't digest it? Apart from keeping the digestive tract happy and healthy, fiber plays an important role in regulating blood sugar levels and hunger. The average adult needs between 25 and 35 grams of fiber per day to maintain good health (*Fiber*, 2012). There are two kinds of fiber:

- **Soluble fiber:** This type dissolves in water and helps the body lower glucose and cholesterol levels. Natural sources of soluble fiber include chia seeds, oatmeal, nuts, lentils, apples, beans, and blueberries.
- **Insoluble fiber:** This type of fiber works by preventing constipation to keep the digestive system in good shape. Fruits with edible skin, such as apples, pears, and grapes, as well as legumes, kale, walnuts, and almonds are all natural sources of insoluble fiber.

The Good of Dietary Fiber

An easy way to up your fiber intake is to replace white rice, bread, and pasta with minimally processed "brown" or whole grain versions. Alternatively, sprinkling some ground flaxseed over breakfast cereals and introducing diced vegetables into stews, soups, and casseroles are viable, low-effort ways of ensuring we are eating enough natural sources of fiber. Fiber does a lot of good in our bodies, including:

- **Promoting regular bowel movements:** Fiber helps to add bulk to the stool, making it easier to pass and promoting regular bowel movements.
- **Lowering cholesterol levels:** Soluble fiber, found in fruits, vegetables, and legumes, binds with bile acids in the stomach, which can help lower cholesterol levels.
- **Helping to control blood sugar levels:** Fiber can slow the absorption of sugar in the bloodstream, which can help control blood sugar levels and reduce the risk of type 2 diabetes.
- **Aiding in weight management:** Fiber is known to make you feel full and satisfied for a longer time, which can be helpful for weight management.
- **Supporting a healthy gut:** Fiber helps feed the beneficial bacteria in the gut, promoting a healthy gut microbiome.

- **Reducing the risk of certain cancers:** Some studies have suggested that a diet high in fiber may reduce the risk of certain types of cancer, such as colon cancer (Masrul & Nindrea, 2019).
- **Supporting heart health:** Eating a diet high in fiber, especially soluble fiber, is associated with a reduced risk of heart disease.

The Bad of Dietary Fiber

While dietary fiber is an important nutrient that plays many vital roles in the body, there are also some potential downsides to consuming too much fiber. When using fiber supplements, such as psyllium or methylcellulose, it becomes very easy to take too much fiber. As a result, we should always try to get our fiber from natural dietary sources first. Some of the main cons of dietary fiber include the following:

- **Digestive discomfort:** Consuming too much fiber can lead to digestive discomforts such as bloating, gas, constipation, and diarrhea.
- **Interference with nutrient absorption:** Consuming too much fiber can interfere with the absorption of certain nutrients, such as iron, zinc, and calcium.

- **Interference with medications:** Consuming too much fiber can interfere with the absorption of certain medications, such as those for diabetes and thyroid disorders (Picco, n.d.).
- **Reduced appetite:** Consuming too much fiber can lead to a feeling of fullness, reducing appetite and making it challenging to consume enough calories.
- **Excessive intake of certain fibers:** Some fibers, such as psyllium husk, can absorb a lot of liquid and expand in the stomach, which can cause blockages in the digestive tract if consumed excessively.

It's crucial to remember that a balanced diet that favors whole foods like fruits, vegetables, whole grains, and legumes over processed foods is advised. According to national health organizations, it is advisable to consume the recommended amount of fiber each day. If you are unsure whether your fiber intake is adequate, speak with a certified dietitian or other healthcare provider to create a custom nutrition plan.

FUNCTIONS OF WATER

Water is essential for all living organisms; it plays several vital roles in the body. Every part of our bodies need water to function optimally. If you can't stand plain old H_2O, you might be relieved to know that tea, orange juice, milk, sparkling water and sports drinks are just as effective in hydrating us (Sweeney, 2021). Keep in mind that these alternative sources of hydration may contain sugars and can add additional calories to your diet plan, so consume them in moderation and try to drink plain water well.

The Good of Water

Every system in the human body needs water, so let's take a closer look at its importance.

- **Regulates body temperature:** Water helps to regulate body temperature by dissipating heat through sweating.
- **Transports nutrients and oxygen:** Water acts as a solvent, helping to transport nutrients and oxygen to cells throughout the body.
- **Removes waste products:** Water helps to flush waste products, such as urea and carbon

dioxide, out of the body through urine and sweat.

- **Lubricates and cushions:** Water acts as a lubricant, helping to protect joints and organs, and cushioning the brain, spinal cord, and other sensitive tissues.
- **Aids in digestion and absorption:** Water helps to break down food and aid in the absorption of nutrients in the gut.
- **Maintains blood pressure:** Water helps to maintain normal blood pressure by regulating blood volume.
- **Encourages skin hydration:** Water helps to keep the skin hydrated, maintaining its elasticity and ability to function as a barrier.
- **Supports physical and cognitive performance:** Adequate hydration is vital for physical and cognitive performance; it can help improve mood, memory, and concentration.

The Bad of Water

While water is essential for good health, there are also some potential downsides to consuming too much water. Some of the main cons of excessive water intake include the following:

- **Hyponatremia:** Consuming too much water can lead to hyponatremia, which occurs when the balance of electrolytes in the body is disrupted, leading to a dangerously low sodium level in the blood. This can cause symptoms such as confusion, nausea, headache, and fatigue, and in severe cases, it can lead to seizures, coma, and even death.
- **Interference with digestion:** Consuming too much water during a meal can dilute stomach acid, interfering with digestion and nutrient absorption.
- **Interference with medications:** Consuming too much water can dilute certain medications and make them less effective.
- **Increased urination:** Consuming too much water can lead to frequent urination, which can be inconvenient or disruptive, particularly when access to a bathroom is limited.

It's important to note that drinking enough water is essential to maintaining good health, and it's important to drink enough water during the day and consume water-rich foods, such as fruits and vegetables, to stay hydrated. The recommended daily water intake varies depending on various factors such as age, sex, activity level, and climate.

FUNCTIONS OF VITAMINS AND MINERALS

Micronutrients are essential to preserve health. According to research, the majority of the vitamins we obtain through food are superior to those found in supplements. Vitamin supplements don't seem to perform as well even when they are synthesized to exactly match the chemical makeup of naturally occurring vitamins (*Vitamin and mineral supplements - what to know*, n.d.). The one exception here is folate. Our bodies seem to absorb the synthetic version better than natural folate found in food. That being said, a healthy, balanced diet generally provides us all the vitamins and minerals we need without the need for supplementation.

The Good of Vitamins and Minerals

Small amounts of vitamins and minerals are required by every cell in the body to carry out a variety of tasks, including:

- **Growth and development:** For healthy growth and development as well as the formation of bones, teeth, and blood cells, vitamins and minerals are crucial.

- **Metabolism:** Vitamins and minerals are essential for metabolism because they aid in the process of turning food into energy and in the body's utilization of that energy. For instance, vitamin B12 is necessary for the breakdown of proteins and fats.
- **Immune system:** Vitamins and minerals help to support the immune system, helping to protect the body from infection and disease. Vitamin C is a great example here, as it aids the immune system in many ways. Megadosing on vitamin C is a common practice among many individuals, but it is not recommended. While it is practically impossible to megadose on dietary vitamin C, historical advocates of supplemental megadosing include Linus Pauling. Pauling won the Nobel Peace Prize in chemistry in 1954 and was of the opinion that megadosing vitamin C can help to increase human lifespan (*Vitamin c megadosage*, 2023). To date, there is not enough credible scientific evidence to support these claims.
- **Hormone production:** Vitamins and minerals are essential for producing hormones, which help regulate bodily functions.
- **Antioxidant function:** The antioxidant properties of vitamins and minerals, in

particular vitamins A, C, and E and the mineral selenium, aid in defending the body against free radical damage.

- **Nervous system function:** Vitamins and minerals are essential for the proper function of the nervous system, helping to transmit nerve impulses and support brain and nerve function.
- **Vision and skin health:** For healthy vision and skin, vitamins and minerals are crucial, especially zinc and vitamin A.
- **Bone health:** For the growth and maintenance of strong bones, vitamins and minerals are crucial, especially calcium and vitamin D.

The Bad of Vitamins and Minerals

There are some potential drawbacks to ingesting too many vitamins and minerals, despite the fact that they are important micronutrients that are crucial for sustaining good health. The following are some of the most significant disadvantages of vitamins and minerals:

- **Toxicity:** Consuming too many specific vitamins and minerals can lead to toxicity, which can cause symptoms such as nausea, vomiting, and even organ damage. For example, excessive intake of vitamin A can cause birth defects and liver damage, while excessive intake of iron can cause damage to the liver and other organs.

- **Interference with medications:** Consuming too many specific vitamins and minerals can interfere with the efficacy of certain medications. For example, high doses of vitamin K can interfere with the effectiveness of blood thinning medications.
- **Interference with nutrient absorption:** Consuming too many specific vitamins and minerals can interfere with the absorption of other nutrients. For example, high calcium doses can interfere with zinc absorption.
- **Nutrient imbalances:** Consuming too many specific vitamins and minerals can lead to imbalances in other nutrients. For example, excessive vitamin C intake can lead to a deficiency in copper.
- **Expensive:** Some vitamin and mineral supplements can be expensive, and consuming too much can be costly and not always necessary.

It's important to note that not all vitamins and minerals are created equal, and it's important to choose nutrient-dense food sources such as fruits, vegetables, whole grains, and lean proteins rather than processed foods.

When and Why to Use Nutritional Supplements

Nutritional supplementation refers to taking additional vitamins, minerals, and other supplements to support overall health and well-being. These supplements can come in various forms, such as pills, capsules, powders, liquids, and bars. They can correct nutrient deficiencies, support special dietary needs, and promote athletic performance, among other things. Let's take a closer look at some of the use cases for nutritional supplements, keeping in mind that supplements are not intended to replace a balanced and healthy diet.

- **Nutrient deficiencies:** Nutritional supplements can help correct nutrient deficiencies that a poor diet, certain medical conditions, or medications may cause. For example, individuals with a vitamin D deficiency may benefit from a vitamin D supplement.
- **Special dietary needs:** Nutritional supplements can help meet the dietary needs of certain populations, such as pregnant women, older adults, or vegetarians.

- **Convenience:** Nutritional supplements can be a convenient way to ensure that you are getting enough of certain nutrients, particularly for individuals who have difficulty consuming certain foods or have limited access to a variety of nutrient-dense foods.
- **Athletic performance:** Some athletes use supplements to enhance physical performance, such as protein powders to help build muscle mass.
- **Medical conditions:** Nutritional supplements can help manage certain medical conditions, such as anemia, osteoporosis, or certain types of cancer.

It's essential to consume a range of nutrient-dense foods as part of a balanced diet to ensure that you obtain all the nutrients you need. Before beginning any supplement routine, it's also crucial to speak with a trained nutritionist or healthcare practitioner because some supplements may interact negatively with certain drugs or pose other hazards.

When we go back to the basics of nutrition, we should realize that a balanced, nutrient-dense diet is essential for maintaining good health. This includes eating various fruits, vegetables, whole grains, lean proteins, and healthy fats while limiting consumption of added sugars, saturated fats, and processed foods. Additionally, it's crucial to stay within your daily calorie needs, drink plenty of water, and follow dietary guidelines and recommendations set by national health organizations.

Another critical aspect of *Going Back to the Basics of Nutrition* is developing a long-term, sustainable approach to healthy eating rather than following fad diets or restrictive eating plans. Consulting a registered dietitian or healthcare professional can help you create a personalized nutrition plan that meets your needs. Ultimately, embracing the basics of nutrition is about making informed decisions about what we eat and developing healthy eating habits that will support our overall well-being.

FOOD DIARY-BASED ACTION

Having a good understanding of basic nutrition is essential to maintain our health in the long run. The food diary can help us make informed meal choices. As in the previous chapters, we'll rate our hunger and satiety levels and inspect our emotions. We'll only introduce one small change here, and that is to reflect on the reason why you choose a particular meal. When completing your food diary reflect on the following questions:

- How can I improve my vitamin and mineral intake without resorting to supplements?
- What positive changes am I noticing on my food journey?
- Has my relationship with food changed? If so, how?

Meal	How Hungry I Felt (scored from 1–10)	Food Consumed	Amount Consumed	How Satiated I Felt (scored from 1–10)	Did I Eat My Emotions? Why Did I Choose These Foods?
Breakfast	4	Oats and fruit smoothie.	Half a portion of oats and a fruit smoothie with banana and apple (prepared at home).	8	I ate because I was hungry. The fruit smoothie was a great way to add fiber to my diet.
Lunch	4	Steak, vegetables, and iced tea.	One sirloin steak, spinach, beets, and an iced tea (prepared by restaurant).	9	I did not eat my emotions. The meal was a good source of protein and vitamins.
Dinner	5	Bacon, eggs, and a fruit smoothie.	Two slices of bacon and two boiled eggs with a blueberry smoothie (prepared at home).	9	I felt a bit homesick and had breakfast for dinner. I tried to keep it healthy, though!

How Do I Feel About My Body Today? Why?			What Exercise Did I Do Today? How Did I Feel Afterwards?		
I feel better about my body every day! I try to keep things healthy and I'm noticing a positive change. I've got more energy!			*I didn't work out today, but I walked to the store instead of driving. It was a 15-minute walk.*		
Breakfast					
Lunch					
Dinner					
How Do I Feel About My Body Today? Why?			**What Exercise Did I Do Today? How Did I Feel Afterwards?**		

7

THE IMPORTANCE OF YOUR BODY COMPOSITION

The ratio of different bodily tissue types, such as muscle, fat, bone, and other tissues, is referred to as body composition. It influences a number of physiological functions and indicates disease risk, making it crucial to general health and fitness. Body composition can be measured in multiple ways, such as through skinfold measurements, bioelectrical impedance analysis (BIA), and dual-energy x-ray absorptiometry (DXA) scans. Don't worry; these measurement methods will be clarified later in the chapter.

Understanding body composition can help individuals make informed decisions about their health and fitness goals. It's important to note that body composition should be considered along with other health indicators, such as blood pressure, cholesterol levels, and blood sugar, to get a complete picture of an individual's health. A healthy body composition can be promoted through regular exercise and healthy eating habits.

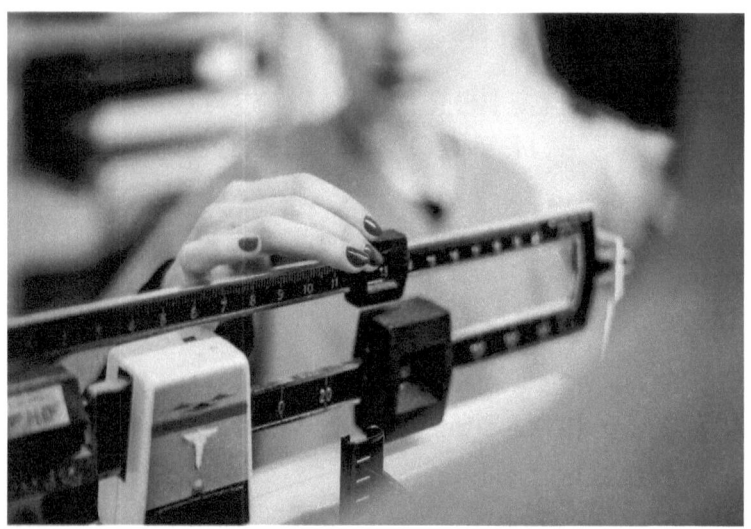

WEIGHT VERSUS BODY COMPOSITION

Whenever people decide to commit to a health and fitness plan, the scale inevitably comes out. We scrutinize the numbers closely and might congratulate ourselves if we manage to lose or gain weight in accordance with our fitness goals. What many people don't realize is that the scale can be quite misleading. Body weight does not accurately reflect overall health and fitness. This is why we rely on body composition to get a more accurate picture of an individual's health by measuring the body's proportion of muscle, fat, and other tissues. The key differences between weight and body composition are as follows:

- Weight is a measure of the amount of mass an individual has. This includes muscle, bone, and fat mass. It is typically measured in pounds or kilograms and can be determined using a scale.
- Body composition measures the relative proportions of muscle, bone, and fat in the body. It is typically measured using skinfold measurements, bioelectrical impedance analysis (BIA), or dual-energy x-ray absorptiometry (DXA).

It is important to note that two people with the same weight may have different body compositions. For example, one person may have a higher muscle mass and a lower body fat percentage. In comparison, another person may have higher body fat and a lower muscle mass percentage. So, body composition is a more accurate measure of overall health and fitness than weight alone. A person with high muscle mass and low body fat is considered healthier and fitter than someone with a high body fat percentage and low muscle mass, even if they have the same weight.

Overall, body composition is a good indicator of whether or not the fat in our bodies falls within a healthy range. This range is determined by factors such as the age and gender of the individual, as indicated in the table below.

Age Range	Percentage Body Fat
20–39	21%–32% for women 8%–18% for men
40–59	23%–33% for women 11%–21% for men
60–79	24%–35% for women 13%–24% for men (Ratini, 2021).

This knowledge is important, as it can mean the difference between developing disease and remaining healthy!

REMOVE DISEASE RISK

A high proportion of body fat, particularly in the abdominal area, has been linked to an increased risk of chronic diseases such as heart disease, diabetes, and certain cancers (Neeland et al., 2015). A healthy body composition with a lower proportion of body fat can help reduce the risk of these diseases. Now that we are a bit more familiar with body composition, the next big question is, "How do you get a healthy body composition?" By paying attention to the following key areas, you'll be able to effectively achieve a healthy body composition:

- **Reduce body fat:** High body fat levels, particularly abdominal fat, are associated with an increased risk of several chronic diseases, such as diabetes, heart disease, and certain cancers. Reducing your body fat percentage can lower your risk of these diseases.
- **Increase muscle mass:** A higher muscle mass is associated with a lower risk of chronic diseases and better overall health outcomes. Increasing your muscle mass can improve your body composition and lower your disease risk.
- **Improve nutrient density:** By consuming nutrient-dense foods and adequate micronutrients, you can support your body composition and reduce your risk of chronic diseases such as obesity, diabetes, heart disease, and cancer.
- **Regular exercise:** Regular physical activity can help you maintain healthy body composition and reduce your risk of chronic diseases. Aim for moderate-intensity aerobic activity or vigorous-intensity aerobic exercise three times per week, along with muscle-strengthening

activities, at least two days a week. By doing so you'll build lean muscle and burn excess fat.

- **Avoid excessive alcohol consumption and smoking:** Both smoking and excessive alcohol are associated with an increased risk of chronic diseases and poor body composition.
- **Maintaining healthy sleep patterns:** Adequate sleep is important for maintaining healthy body composition and reducing the risk of chronic diseases. Aim for seven to nine hours of sleep per night, and establish a consistent sleep schedule.

PHYSICAL PERFORMANCE

The human body has more than 600 muscles (Garrick, 2017). These muscles are vital to helping us move, breathe, talk, and circulate blood throughout the body. Keeping our muscles healthy is therefore crucial to maintaining overall health. A higher proportion of muscle in the body can improve physical performance, as muscle is more metabolically active than fat and can help boost energy levels. When working towards improving our physical performance, it is crucial to focus on the following:

- **Increase muscle mass:** A higher muscle mass is associated with improved physical performance, such as increased strength and power. By increasing your muscle mass, you can improve your overall physical performance.
- **Improve cardiovascular fitness:** A higher cardiovascular fitness level is associated with improved physical performance. By engaging in regular aerobic exercise, you can improve your cardiovascular and physical fitness.
- **Proper rest and recovery:** Adequate rest and recovery are essential for physical performance, as it allows the body to repair and rebuild muscle tissue, replenish energy stores, and reduce the risk of injury.
- **Adequate hydration:** Staying hydrated is essential for physical performance, as it allows the body to maintain an optimal temperature, support muscle, and joint function, and flush out waste products.

WEIGHT MANAGEMENT

Maintaining a healthy body composition naturally helps with weight management, as muscle burns more calories than fat and can help boost metabolism. If weight management is one of your health goals, it is important to pay attention to the following key areas:

- **Identifying areas of concern:** Body composition analysis can provide information on the body's fat, muscle, and bone proportion. This information can help identify areas of concern, such as high body fat levels, which may contribute to weight gain.
- **Setting realistic goals:** By understanding your body composition, you can set realistic weight management goals. For example, if you have a high muscle mass and a low body fat percentage, your goal may be to maintain your current weight rather than lose weight.
- **Tracking progress:** Body composition analysis can track progress over time and monitor changes in muscle mass, body fat, and overall weight. This can help you determine the effectiveness of your weight management plan and make adjustments as needed.
- **Adjusting diet and exercise:** By understanding your body composition, you can change your diet and exercise plan to target specific areas. For example, suppose you have a high body fat percentage. In that case, you may want to focus on reducing calories and increasing physical

activity. In contrast, you may want to focus on boosting protein intake and resistance training if you have a low muscle mass.

- **Identifying underlying issues:** Body composition analysis can also reveal underlying health issues contributing to weight gain or difficulty with weight management, such as hormonal imbalances or metabolic disorders. By identifying these underlying issues, you can address them and develop a more effective weight management plan.
- **Tailoring a specific plan:** Body composition analysis can provide information that can help tailor a detailed plan for weight management. For example, suppose you have a high body fat percentage. In that case, you may need to focus on reducing calorie intake, increasing physical activity, and strength training to increase muscle mass and protein intake. To increase muscle mass, you may need to focus on increasing your calorie intake, protein intake, and resistance training.

Knowing your body composition can give you useful information that can help you manage your weight by allowing you to pinpoint problem areas, set reasonable goals, monitor your progress, make necessary dietary and exercise adjustments, identify underlying problems, and create a customized plan to reach your weight management objectives. Overall, knowing your body composition is extremely useful for achieving your health goals.

HOW TO MEASURE TO FIND OUT WHAT YOUR BODY COMPOSITION IS

For those curious about finding out their body composition, there are five different ways to go about this. Each method varies in complexity and accuracy but will give individuals a good insight into their body fat percentage. Let's take a brief look at each of these tests.

Skinfold Test

These tests are the most basic way to measure the amount of body fat in an individual. Due to its simplicity, the skinfold test tends to be the least accurate of the available methods (Satrazemis, 2021).

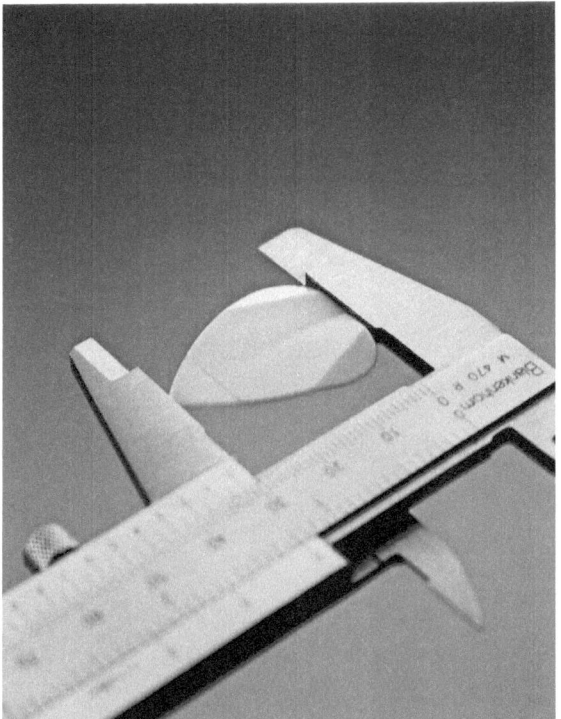

With skinfold tests, calipers are used to gently pinch select areas of the body (such as the chest, thighs, and abdomen). The thickness of the skinfold is then measured. The measurements are then combined with other data (the person's age and gender) into a specific formula to obtain the body fat estimate. It is a simple and straightforward process, but there are some limitations.

One of the biggest limitations of skinfold tests is that they can only measure subcutaneous fat, i.e., fat under the skin. Therefore, it is not a full-body assessment.

Everyone's genetic makeup differs, so not everyone will store fat in the same way. Also, skinfold tests allow a lot of room for human error to slip in during measuring. Gyms, fitness centers, and health professionals may offer skinfold tests, but be aware that the results and costs thereof may vary.

The Jackson–Pollock skinfold formula is commonly used to work out body fat percentage. The math is pretty straightforward, and you'll only need to measure the skinfolds at three sites. The measurement sites and formula differ for men and women, as explained in the table below.

Formula Used	Measurement Site (Measured in millimeters)
Women: • Add your skinfold measurements together to obtain Value A. • Take Value A and multiply it with itself to obtain Value B (square Value A). • Substitute values obtained into the formula below to calculate BD (body density). BD = 1.0994921 − (0.0009929 x Value A) + (0.0000023 x Value B) − (0.0001392 x age) • Substitute BD into the formula below to calculate BFP (body fat percentage). BFP = (495 / BD) − 450	• **Triceps:** Pinch the skin on the back of your arm midway between the elbow and the shoulder. • **Thigh:** Halfway between the top of your kneecap and the top of your front thigh, pinch the skin vertically. • **Suprailiac measurement:** On the front of your right hip, pinch the skin in a diagonal direction just above the bony protrusion (the iliac crest).
Men: • Add your skinfold measurements together to obtain Value A. • Take Value A and multiply it with itself to obtain Value B (square Value A). • Substitute values obtained into the formula below to calculate BD (body density). BD = 1.10938 − (0.0008267 x Value A) + (0.0000016 x Value B) − (0.0002574 x age) • Substitute BD into the formula below to calculate BFP (body fat percentage). BFP = (495 / BD) − 450	• **Pectoral:** Pinch a diagonal skinfold midway between your right nipple and armpit. • **Abdominal:** One inch to the right of your belly button, pinch the skin vertically. • **Thigh:** Halfway between the top of your kneecap and the top of your front thigh, pinch the skin vertically (Moore, 2021).

Bioelectrical Impedance Analysis (BIA)

This test is a bit more complicated and makes use of a low electric current to estimate fat mass. The mechanics behind this test are quite ingenious. Since electricity can travel through water, and all our bodily tissues contain varying amounts of it, the flow of the electric current is affected by the conductivity of our tissues. Since muscle holds more water than fat, it will be more conductive and create less resistance in the current. This data is then fed into an algorithm that will calculate the body fat percentage of the individual.

As fascinating as BIA tools can be, there is one big limitation. Our hydration status can impact the accuracy of the measurements. In addition to this, exercise or having a meal before taking the test can also impact its accuracy. That being said, the results are usually pretty accurate. The margin of error usually hovers between three and eight percent (Burns et al., 2019). Home scales using the technology may have a higher margin of error, but they still provide a fairly accurate guess of body fat percentage.

Underwater Weighing

Also called hydrostatic weighing, this method makes use of our body weight on land and in water with additional data (the amount of water displaced) to calculate fat percentage. It is a method that has its roots in Archimedes' principle. Simply put, the volume of water displaced is equal to the volume of the submerged object. This makes the Archimedes principle super useful for calculating the density of something. Since muscle is denser than fat, it will displace less water.

According to this principle, a person with more muscle mass will therefore weigh more underwater than someone who has a high percentage of body fat (Lee & Gallagher, 2008).

The individual that is being weighed is required to exhale during the test, as any air in the lungs can impact the accuracy of the measurement. The test is usually repeated three times, and the average is then calculated and presented as the percentage of body fat. That being said, the test is remarkably accurate, with an error margin of less than three percent (*Body Fat Testing through Underwater Weighing*, n.d.).

One of the biggest limitations of this test is that it is only offered by select fitness companies, so it might not be an accessible option for everyone.

Air Displacement (BodPod)

This measurement technique has a lot in common with hydrostatic weighing, save for one crucial change: an egg-shaped pod replaces the water. If you are claustrophobic, perhaps it would be best to give this method a skip, as it requires you to be seated in an enclosed pod. From there, a mechanical diaphragm creates small changes to the volume inside the pod and collects the resulting data. This data is combined with the individual's weight, gender, age, and height to calculate their fat percentage. It is pretty much the Archimedes' principle applied to air. Since fat is less dense than muscle, the results are as accurate as hydrostatic weighing (Lowry & Tomiyama, 2015). Once again, the only limitation to this method would be that it is only offered at select institutions, so it might not be accessible to everyone.

DEXA Scan

The DEXA scan (alternatively called a DXA scan) differs significantly from the aforementioned methods. Not only is it the most accurate body composition analysis tool available, but it gives us information that the other methods can't. This technique employs X-ray technology to differentiate between subcutaneous and visceral fat, as well as muscle imbalances and bone density! It is truly a comprehensive tool for body composition analysis. Only select institutions offer DEXA scans, so they might not be accessible to everyone.

The five methods mentioned above are typically used in professional settings, but methods to determine your body composition at home do exist. Two popular measurement techniques at home are:

- **Body Measurement Tape:** Measuring the circumferences of different body parts, such as the waist, hips, and thighs, can be used to estimate body fat percentage.
- **At-Home Scales:** Some at-home scales use bioelectrical impedance analysis (BIA) to estimate body fat percentage.

It's important to remember that self-measurement methods can be less accurate than professional methods, such as a dual-energy X-ray absorptiometry (DXA) scan. Also, before beginning any self-measurement methods, consult a healthcare professional and understand the results and how they relate to health and fitness goals.

WHY BODY COMPOSITION MEASUREMENT IS BETTER THAN BODY MASS INDEX (BMI)

Chances are that you'd be familiar with the term "BMI" or body mass index. You might even know what your BMI is. Perhaps you worked fervently to get your BMI down from that scary 30 that carries the "obese" brand with it. The thing is, BMI is to body composition what analog TV is to streaming services: Dated and limited. Just like the analog TVs of old only showed a black-and-white picture, BMI only gives us limited information. It paints a picture of our body mass relative to our height. It is not an indicator of how much body fat or muscle an individual has (Carson, 2019). Body composition, by stark contrast, gives us a much clearer picture. This method is considered to be a more accurate way to assess overall health and fitness compared to BMI for several reasons:

- **BMI cannot differentiate between muscle and fat:** BMI is calculated based on weight and height and does not consider the body's muscle, fat, and other tissue proportion. This means that a person with a high ratio of muscle mass may be classified as overweight or obese based on their BMI, even though they have a healthy body composition.
- **BMI does not account for body shape:** BMI does not consider the distribution of fat in the body, which can affect disease risk. For example, a person with a high proportion of abdominal fat may be at an increased risk of chronic diseases even if their BMI is within a healthy range.
- **Athletes and older adults:** BMI is not as accurate for specific populations, such as athletes and older adults. Athletes have a higher proportion of muscle mass and may be

classified as overweight or obese based on their BMI, even though they have a healthy body composition. Similarly, older adults may have a lower proportion of muscle mass and a higher proportion of body fat, which can affect their health and fitness, but their BMI may not reflect this.

Body composition is significant in general health and fitness because it influences a variety of physiological functions and predicts illness risk. Physical performance, weight management, and beauty may all be enhanced by having a healthy body composition. Body composition is defined as having a healthy proportion of fat relative to muscle mass. Please understand that fat is not the enemy. Our bodies need fat, but too much or too little of it can be harmful. Knowing one's body composition can assist us in identifying and addressing potential health problems, as well as making educated decisions around our fitness and health objectives. It's important to note that body composition should be considered along with other health indicators, such as blood pressure, cholesterol levels, and blood sugar, to get a complete picture of an individual's health. A healthy body composition can be promoted through regular exercise and healthy eating habits.

FOOD DIARY-BASED ACTION

Having a good understanding of your body composition can only make your health and fitness goals more attainable. When we know how much (or how little) fat and muscle we have, adjusting our diets accordingly becomes a much easier task. In this chapter's food diary activity, we won't be making any changes, however, you are encouraged to reflect on the following questions when completing your entry:

- Do I know my body composition? If not, it is recommended to find out. Even a simple skin fold test can provide us with a good starting point.
- What changes should I make to my diet that will suit my body and health goals?
- Did finding out my body composition impact my relationship with food? If so, how?

Meal	How Hungry I Felt (scored from 1–10)	Food Consumed	Amount Consumed	How Satiated I Felt (scored from 1–10)	Did I Eat My Emotions? Why Did I Choose These Foods?
Breakfast	4	Cheesy omelets and coffee.	One large, cheesy omelet (prepared at home), and a coffee with sugar and milk.	8	I ate because I was hungry and focused more on proteins this morning.
Lunch	-	-	-	-	Skipped lunch. Had my body composition analyzed and did not have time to eat afterwards.
Dinner	2	Roast chicken and vegetables.	Roast chicken (drumstick and wing) with cauliflower and sweet potato.	9	I was a bit upset after learning how much fat I carried on my body, but I can proudly say I did not eat my emotions!

How Do I Feel About My Body Today? Why?			What Exercise Did I Do Today? How Did I Feel Afterwards?		
I felt a bit awkward after finding out what my body composition is, but I'm determined to reduce my belly fat!			*I focused on strength-training exercises today. Did a 30-minute workout with light weights. Felt surprisingly energetic afterwards!*		
Breakfast					
Lunch					
Dinner					
How Do I Feel About My Body Today? Why?			What Exercise Did I Do Today? How Did I Feel Afterwards?		

8

UNDERSTANDING THE IMPACT OF UNKNOWN FOOD EFFECTS ON YOUR BODY

Unknown food effects refer to food-related issues that people may not be aware of, such as food allergies, intolerances, sensitivities, nutrient deficiencies, and reactions to additives and preservatives. These issues can be hard to identify and diagnose and can cause a range of mild to severe symptoms that can negatively impact overall health. These issues can be caused by various factors, such as genetics, lifestyle, and exposure to certain substances, and can be triggered by consuming certain foods.

Food sensitivities or symptoms can be caused by an immune system reaction to certain foods, which can be challenging to pinpoint without proper testing. Suppose you suspect that you may have an unknown food sensitivity or allergy. In that case, it's important to consult with a healthcare professional who can help you determine the best course of action. This may include an elimination diet, which involves removing certain foods from your diet for some time and then gradually reintroducing them to see which foods trigger symptoms. Other diagnostic tests that identify food sensitivities include blood tests, skin prick tests, and oral food challenges. It's important to note that food sensitivities and allergies are different, and treatment will vary depending on the underlying condition. Common food allergens include peanuts, tree nuts, milk, eggs, and shellfish.

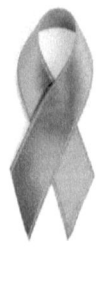

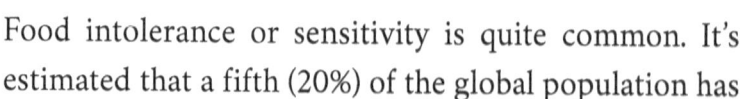

Food intolerance or sensitivity is quite common. It's estimated that a fifth (20%) of the global population has a food intolerance of some kind (Zopf et al., 2009). More disturbingly, it seems that food intolerances and sensitivities may be on the rise. This might be due to changes in the way our food is manufactured, but it is just as likely that a complex interplay between environmental, social, economical, and genetic factors is responsible (Hadley, 2006). Simply put, the way we eat can potentially trigger allergies and sensitivities.

Take the humble peanut as an example. Peanut allergies in the United States just about doubled from 1997 to 2002 (Venter et al., 2006). Peanuts are commonly dry roasted, a practice that increases their allergenicity when compared to boiling or frying (Chung et al., 2003). Interestingly, researchers found that in China and many African countries where peanuts are commonly boiled or fried, very low rates of peanut allergies are found when compared to the United States. This suggests that our relationship with food, especially how and when a food item is introduced into our diets, plays a role in the development of food allergies and sensitivities. That being said, let's take a closer look at food allergies and sensitivities.

FOOD ALLERGIES MAY HINDER FOOD SELECTION

Food allergies occur when the immune system mistakenly identifies a particular food as harmful and reacts to it. Allergies are particularly common among children, and it is believed that one child in every 13 suffers from food allergies (*Food allergy versus food intolerance*, n.d.). Food allergy reactions can be life-threatening, placing 200,000 Americans every year in the emergency room (*Facts and statistics*, n.d.).

How can you tell whether anything you ate triggered an allergic reaction? Symptoms of a food allergy often appear within minutes after swallowing the food item. Common symptoms to be on the lookout for include:

- rash or hives
- swelling of the face, throat, or eyes
- nausea
- diarrhea
- stomach pain
- feeling lightheaded or dizzy
- vomiting

In the worst-case scenario, an individual with a food allergy may experience anaphylaxis. This is a severe allergic reaction that can cause the airways to constrict, leading to difficulty breathing and a drop in blood pressure. Shock, vomiting, nausea, and a skin rash may accompany this reaction (*Anaphylaxis - symptoms and causes*, 2021). Anaphylaxis can be life-threatening and requires immediate medical attention. This reaction can occur within moments of ingesting a food item.

Remember the honeydew melon incident I told you about in Chapter 5? That was a case of anaphylaxis. The medical staff had to use epinephrine injections and other emergency treatments to curb and reverse the reaction. It was a truly scary experience, but I'll share the important tip the doctor shared with me. He said, "Whenever a reaction like this happens, your best bet is to stay calm." The doctor explained that the minute we panic, the reaction intensifies. By staying calm as best we can, we are giving ourselves and the medical staff treating us a fighting chance.

Other effects food allergies have on us may include:

- **Weight loss or weight gain:** Food allergies can cause abdominal discomfort, diarrhea, and vomiting, making it challenging to maintain a healthy diet and stick to a regular meal schedule. This can lead to weight loss or weight gain over time.

- **Nutrient deficiencies:** Food allergies can lead to avoiding certain foods, which can lead to nutrient deficiencies. For example, if someone is allergic to peanuts, they may avoid all foods containing peanuts, which can limit their intake of essential nutrients.
- **Dehydration:** Intestinal discomfort caused by food allergies can lead to diarrhea and dehydration, which can cause muscle cramps and fatigue. This can make it challenging to stick to an exercise plan and negatively impact physical performance.
- **Inflammation:** Food allergies can cause an immune response which leads to inflammation in the body. This can lead to chronic inflammation, which can contribute to weight gain, muscle loss, and overall body composition changes.
- **Hormonal imbalances:** Food allergies can cause an increase in stress hormones such as cortisol, leading to weight gain, muscle loss, and overall body composition changes.

IT MIGHT BE FOOD INTOLERANCE

Food intolerances occur when the body cannot properly digest or absorb certain foods. Symptoms can range from mild, such as bloating or diarrhea, to severe, such as migraines or chronic fatigue. It is important to note that food intolerance or sensitivity is not the same thing as a food allergy. The former mainly involves our digestive system, while the latter elicits an immune response. Some specific food intolerances include lactose, gluten, histamine, caffeine, artificial sweeteners, coloring agents, and flavorings (*Food allergy versus food intolerance*, n.d.). Food intolerance can have the following effects on our bodies:

- **Weight gain:** Food intolerance can cause bloating, gas, and abdominal discomfort, making it challenging to stick to a healthy diet and exercise plan. This can eventually lead to weight gain.
- **Nutrient deficiencies:** Food intolerances can lead to the avoidance of certain foods, leading to nutrient deficiencies. For example, if someone is intolerant to lactose, they may avoid dairy products, which are a good source of calcium and vitamin D.
- **Dehydration:** Intestinal discomfort caused by a food intolerance can lead to diarrhea and dehydration, which can cause muscle cramps and fatigue. This can make it difficult to stick to an exercise plan and negatively impact physical performance.

- **Inflammation:** An immunological reaction brought on by food intolerance might result in inflammation throughout the body. Chronic inflammation may result from this, and chronic inflammation has been linked to weight gain, muscle loss, and changes in general body composition (*Is a Food Allergy Causing You Inflammation?*, 2018).
- **Hormonal imbalances:** A rise in stress hormones like cortisol brought on by food intolerances can result in weight gain, muscle loss, and general changes in body composition (Mahtani, 2020).

It's important to note that food intolerance affects each person differently, and the severity of symptoms can vary widely. If you suspect you have a food intolerance, it's important to consult a healthcare professional to determine the best course of action.

HIDDEN FOOD SENSITIVITIES

Some people may be sensitive to certain foods they eat on a regular basis but are unaware of it. This can be due to chronic health issues masking symptoms such as headaches, joint pain, skin problems, and fatigue. Hidden food sensitivities can contribute to:

- **Weight gain or weight loss:** Hidden food sensitivities can cause abdominal discomfort, diarrhea, and other digestive issues, making it difficult to maintain a healthy diet and stick to a regular meal schedule. This can lead to weight loss or weight gain over time.
- **Nutrient deficiencies:** Hidden food sensitivities can lead to avoiding certain foods, leading to nutrient deficiencies. For example, if someone is sensitive to gluten, they may prevent gluten-containing foods, limiting their intake of essential nutrients.
- **Dehydration:** Intestinal discomfort caused by hidden food sensitivities can lead to diarrhea and dehydration, which can cause muscle cramps and fatigue. This can make it difficult to stick to an exercise plan and negatively impact physical performance.
- Inflammation: Hidden food sensitivities may trigger an immunological response that results in bodily inflammation. Chronic inflammation brought on by this may result in weight gain, muscle loss, and general changes in body

composition (*Is a food allergy causing you inflammation?*, 2018).

- **Hormonal imbalances:** Unidentified food sensitivities can raise stress hormones like cortisol, which can result in weight gain, muscle loss, and changes to general body composition (Mahtani, 2020).
- Fatigue: Hidden food sensitivities can cause fatigue, which can make it difficult to stick to an exercise plan and can negatively impact physical performance (*Food allergies and fatigue*, n.d.).

Hidden food sensitivities are more complex to detect than allergies or intolerances. It's important to consult a healthcare professional to determine the best course of action. Identifying and eliminating the specific foods causing the sensitivity can help alleviate symptoms and improve overall health and body composition.

YOU COULD BE NUTRIENT DEFICIENT

A diet deficient in nutrients can result in a number of unpleasant symptoms. These symptoms are the body's way of telling us that something is not right, that you may be experiencing possible vitamin and mineral shortages. The eight common signs that you might have a nutrient deficiency include the following:

- Brittle nails and hair: There are many causes for brittle nails and hair, but the most common cause is a biotin (vitamin B7) deficiency (Biotin, n.d.). Egg yolks, fish, dairy, nuts, seeds, cauliflower, and bananas are among the foods high in biotin and are normally included in a healthy diet.
- Cracks in your mouth corners or mouth ulcers: An inadequate intake of specific vitamins or minerals may be partially responsible for lesions in and around the mouth. For instance, canker sores, often known as mouth ulcers, are frequently brought on by an iron or B vitamin deficiency (*Canker sore - symptoms and causes*, n.d.).
- **Bleeding gums:** If you are not brushing too hard, then bleeding gums could point to a vitamin C deficiency. Diets low in vitamin C in the long run might result in tooth loss (Institute of Medicine, 2000). So, it's extra important to eat your fruits and vegetables to keep your smile healthy!
- **Poor night vision:** A diet lacking in nutrients might occasionally result in eyesight issues.

Inadequate vitamin A intake, for example, is frequently linked to night blindness, a condition that impairs vision in low light or at night.

- **Dandruff and scaly patches:** A diet lacking in nutrients is one of the numerous potential causes of dandruff and scaly patches (seborrheic dermatitis). Low blood levels of zinc, niacin (vitamin B3), riboflavin (vitamin B2), and pyridoxine (vitamin B6), for example, are thought to contribute to the development of the condition (Petre, 2019).

- **Hair loss or excessive shedding:** This is a very common symptom and points to a possible deficiency in several vitamins and minerals including iron, vitamin B7 and zinc.

- **Bumps on the skin:** Red or white bumps on the skin (also called Keratosis pilaris) is a condition that is not yet fully understood. It is believed that a diet low in vitamin A and C may contribute to the development thereof (Institute of Medicine, 2000).

- **Restless leg syndrome:** This is a condition where one might experience unpleasant sensations in the legs as well as the urge to move them. The cause of the condition is not fully understood but it is believed that a link between restless leg syndrome and an iron deficiency exists (Trenkwalder et al., 2008).

Not getting enough of certain nutrients from food, such as vitamin D, iron, or omega-3 fatty acids, can lead to deficiencies that can negatively impact overall health in several ways, including:

- **Weight loss:** Muscle loss leads to weight loss. For example, a protein deficiency can lead to muscle loss, which can cause weight loss and changes in muscle mass.
- **Fatigue:** This can make it difficult to stick to an exercise plan and negatively impacts physical performance. For example, an iron deficiency can cause fatigue and make it difficult to perform physical activities.
- Weakness: Nutrient deficiencies can cause weakness, making it difficult to perform physical activities. For example, a deficiency in Vitamin D can cause weakness and muscle pain (*Vitamin D deficiency*, n.d.).
- **Hormonal imbalances:** Hormonal imbalances can lead to weight gain, muscle loss, and overall body composition changes.
- **Chronic inflammation:** Deficiencies can cause chronic inflammation, which can contribute to

weight gain, muscle loss, and overall body composition changes.

It's important to note that nutrient deficiencies can cause a range of symptoms that can vary from person to person. Consult a healthcare professional to determine the best course of action and to prevent nutrient deficiencies. It's important to have a well-balanced diet that includes a variety of nutrient-dense foods and to take dietary supplements as necessary.

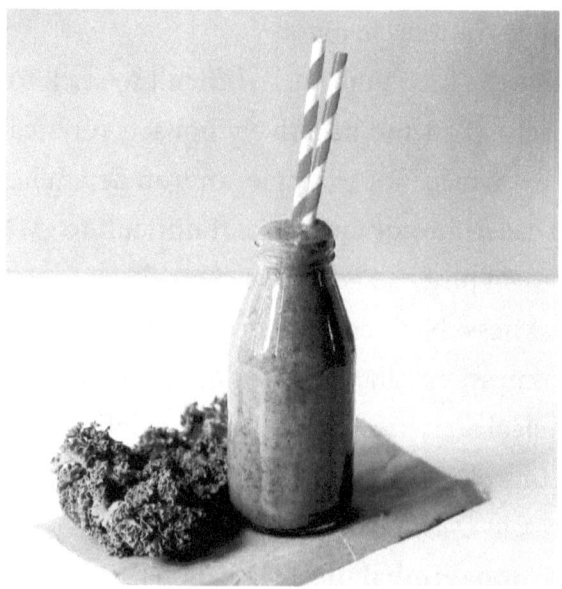

It May Be Additives and Preservatives

Some people may be sensitive to certain additives and preservatives in food, such as sulfites or MSG, which can cause symptoms such as headaches and asthma. It's important to be vigilant about monitoring one's health, pay attention to any signs related to food consumption, and seek professional help if necessary.

THE IMPORTANCE OF A HEALTHY GUT

The majority of us are aware of the gut's fundamental function and that it is home to helpful microorganisms. These bacteria, sometimes referred to as "gut flora," support the digestive process. The species of gut flora are numerous, but not all of them are considered "good bacteria." Like everything else in nature, a delicate balance between good and harmful bacteria exists. However, when this equilibrium is thrown off and the bad gut flora begin to dominate, it may have an impact on our general health (*Gut health: why is it important?*, 2022). A healthy gut essentially means maintaining that delicate balance! When we have a healthy gut, we may benefit from the following:

- **Improved digestion:** A healthy gut can help to break down and absorb nutrients from food more effectively.
- **Boosted immune system:** The gut is home to 70% of the immune system (Vighi et al., 2008). A strong immune system is correlated with a healthy gut.
- **Reduced inflammation:** A healthy gut can help reduce inflammation throughout the body, lowering the risk of chronic diseases such as heart disease and diabetes.
- **Improved mental health:** The gut and brain are connected through the gut-brain axis, and a healthy gut can help to improve mood and reduce anxiety and depression.
- **Weight management:** A healthy gut can help control cravings, regulate appetite and promote weight loss.
- **Better skin health:** A healthy gut can help improve the skin's condition by reducing inflammation, preventing acne, and promoting a clear complexion.
- **Better nutrient absorption:** A healthy gut can help to absorb more nutrients from the food you eat, which can help to prevent nutrient deficiencies.

- **Improved regularity:** A healthy gut can help to promote regular bowel movements and prevent constipation.

Tips to Maintain a Healthy Gut

The easy-to-apply tips below will help us take care of the helpful bacteria, encouraging a healthy gut.

- Consume a diet rich in whole grains, fruits, and vegetables to encourage a healthy gut.
- Include fermented foods in your diet, such as yogurt, kefir, sauerkraut, and kimchi, as they contain beneficial bacteria that can help promote the growth of good bacteria in the gut.
- Avoid processed foods and excessive sugar, as they can disrupt the balance of bacteria in the gut.
- Stay hydrated by drinking plenty of water.
- Consider taking a probiotic supplement, which can help to replenish the good bacteria in the gut.
- Exercise regularly as it helps in maintaining a healthy gut.
- Minimize the use of antibiotics, as they can kill off beneficial bacteria in the gut.

- Manage stress levels, as chronic stress can disrupt the balance of bacteria in the gut.

FOOD DIARY-BASED ACTION

Food intolerances, allergies, and sensitivities can make reaching our health goals a bit more challenging, especially when these conditions go undiagnosed. We won't be making any changes to this chapter's food diary entry, but as you complete the activity ask yourself the following:

- Does my diet encourage a healthy gut? If not, how can I apply the *Tips to Maintain a Healthy Gut* to my eating plan?
- Do I have any symptoms of nutrient deficiency? If so, how will I go about remedying it?
- Do I have or suspect any food allergies or sensitivities? If so, how does that impact my relationship with food?

Meal	How Hungry I Felt (scored from 1–10)	Food Consumed	Amount Consumed	How Satiated I Felt (scored from 1–10)	Did I Eat My Emotions? Why Did I Choose These Foods?
Breakfast	3	Fruit bowl with yogurt.	Fruit bowl containing banana, blueberries, strawberry, and kiwi topped with probiotic yogurt.	7	I was hungry. The fruit bowl was a great way to add vitamins and probiotics to my diet.
Lunch	4	Barbeque chicken and roast vegetables.	Had a barbecued chicken thigh with sweet corn, brussel sprouts, and sweet potato (prepared at home).	9	Trying to prepare the majority of my meals at home to make them as healthy as possible, without sacrificing taste.
Dinner	5	Fruit bowl with probiotic yogurt.	Fruit bowl with banana, raspberry, strawberry, blackberry, and kiwi topped with probiotic yogurt.	9	I was fairly full from lunch and opted for something light and nutrient dense.

How Do I Feel About My Body Today? Why?	What Exercise Did I Do Today? How Did I Feel Afterwards?
My complexion looks brighter today! Must be all the fruit and veg that I've been adding to my diet over the last few weeks!	*I went for a swim and a walk at the beach today. Spent about 30 minutes in the water and walked a mile along the coast at a brisk pace. I'm a bit tired, but I feel great!*

Breakfast					
Lunch					
Dinner					

How Do I Feel About My Body Today? Why?	What Exercise Did I Do Today? How Did I Feel Afterwards?

9

DESIGN A HEALTHY MEAL PLAN

D esigning a healthy meal plan is about creating a structured plan that outlines the types and amounts of foods an individual should eat. Bear in mind that these foods should meet an individual's nutritional needs and aid in achieving health goals. A healthy meal plan should be based on nutrient-dense whole foods, balanced macronutrients, and appropriate portions. These plans are typically tailored to an individual's unique needs, taking factors such as age, activity levels, sex, health status, dietary restrictions and allergies or food sensitivities into account. Healthy meal plans should also take into account personal preferences and cultural food habits. That way we'll be able to make sustainable long-term changes to the way we eat. It may sound a little bit intimidating at first, but after this chapter you'll have a better understanding of what a healthy meal plan is.

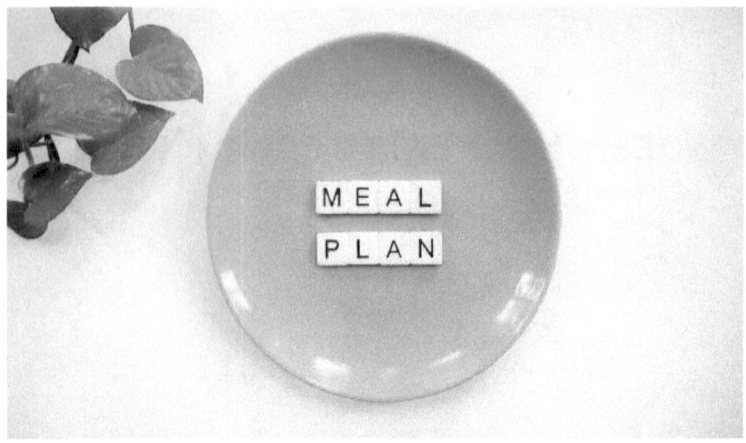

When designing a healthy meal plan, focusing on nutrient-dense whole foods, such as fruits, vegetables, whole grains, lean proteins, and healthy fats, is essential. These foods provide essential nutrients and are more satiating than processed foods. It's also important to include balanced macronutrients, such as carbohydrates, proteins, and healthy fats, in each meal. This will help an individual feel full and satisfied for extended periods.

All of this information might feel a bit overwhelming, so here's an important tip to keep in mind: Make minor adjustments to your meal plan over time rather than trying to make drastic changes all at once. It's also advisable to consult with a healthcare professional, such as a dietitian or nutritionist, to determine the specific nutrient needs and to provide personalized guidance in creating a healthy meal plan. Remember that a healthy meal plan is not a one-size-fits-all solution and that specific nutritional needs may vary depending on an individual's unique health needs.

CREATING A SYSTEMATIC MEAL PLAN FOR ALL

It's an open secret that a healthy eater is an organized one. Now, before you run for the hills, thinking that meal planning is not your thing, I encourage you to consider the benefits of the practice. Yes, you'll need to invest some time into your meal plan, but a well-constructed meal plan can help with the following:

- **Saving time:** One of barriers to healthy eating is a lack of time (Freeman, n.d.). By deciding ahead of time what we'll eat, we still get to enjoy healthy, hearty meals without having to rely on convenience foods.
- **Can reduce stress:** In our busy, modern lives meal planning gives us some breathing room, because our meals are already taken care of.
- **Makes it easier to eat healthily:** Meal planning provides you the power to be deliberate about

incorporating healthy foods into meals and snacks.

- **Saves money:** Meal planning is a budget-friendly activity as we only need to buy the food items we need. You'll be surprised with how much you can save on a healthy meal plan!

Most importantly, meal planning puts the power of making healthy and informed food choices back into your hands! There are many other benefits to meal planning, but I'm sure you've got the gist of it. Taking the time once a week to plan meals that align with your health goals and food preferences will pay off handsomely in the long run. When you go about your meal planning, make sure to focus on the following:

- **Assess your nutrient needs:** Determine your calorie needs and the recommended intake of macronutrients (carbohydrates, proteins, and fats) and micronutrients (vitamins and minerals) based on your age, sex, activity level, and health status.
- **Focus on whole foods:** Include a variety of whole, unprocessed foods in your meal plans, such as fruits, vegetables, whole grains, lean proteins, and healthy fats. These foods provide

essential nutrients and are more satiating than processed foods.

- **Plan your meals and snacks:** Plan your meals and snacks to ensure that you have the necessary ingredients and avoid last-minute decisions that may lead to unhealthy choices.
- **Include a balance of macronutrients:** Include a balance of carbohydrates, proteins, and healthy fats in each meal. This will help you to feel full and satisfied for extended periods.
- **Include a variety of colors:** Incorporate various colors in your meals to ensure you get a wide range of nutrients.
- **Control portion sizes:** Be aware of portion sizes and use measuring cups or a food scale to help ensure that you are not overeating.
- **Incorporate physical activity:** Physical activity is essential to a healthy lifestyle. Make sure to include at least 30 minutes of moderate-intensity physical activity most days of the week.
- **Consider any food allergies, sensitivities, or restrictions:** Adjust your meal plan accordingly if you have any food allergies, sensitivities, or restrictions.

- **Make minor adjustments:** Make small adjustments to your meal plan over time rather than trying to make drastic changes all at once.
- **Consult with a healthcare professional:** Consult with a healthcare professional, such as a dietitian or nutritionist, to determine your specific nutrient needs and for personalized guidance in creating a healthy meal plan.

SELECTION OF A MEAL PLAN

When it comes to choosing a meal plan, it is always advised to pick one that can be tailored to your personal needs. Speak with your healthcare provider before starting a new meal plan or weight-loss program. It is also a good idea to discuss any medical conditions you have or medications that you are taking with your doctor. Your healthcare provider can help you select the meal plan that is the safest and best suited for you. When deciding on a meal plan, consider the following:

- **Past diets:** What did you like or dislike about a past diet you tried? How did these eating plans make you feel on a physical and emotional level? Was it hard to follow the eating plan?

- **Preferences:** Do you prefer to do your own thing, or do you like the support group atmosphere? If you like support groups, consider if online support or in-person meetings are more your speed.
- **The budget:** Some eating plans will require you to purchase additional supplements or specific produce (*Weight loss: choosing a diet that's right for you,* 2018). For an eating plan to be sustainable, it will need to fit your budget.

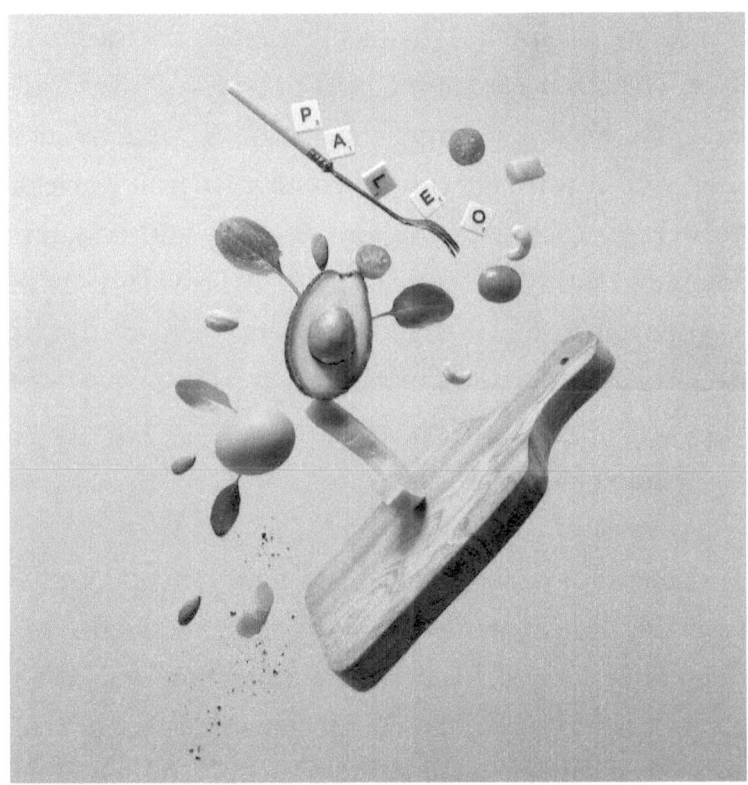

By considering these factors, you'll be able to better select a meal plan that fits into your lifestyle. That being said, let's take a closer look at the different eating plans that promote overall health.

- **Balanced diet:**

This diet includes a balance of macronutrients (carbohydrates, proteins, and fats) and micronutrients (vitamins and minerals). It consists of various foods from all food groups, such as fruits, vegetables, whole grains, lean proteins, and healthy fats. No foods are off-limits here. The balanced diet typically provides all the nutrients we need and supplementation is usually not needed. If you are not sure where to start, or if you lean heavily on processed foods for your daily nutrition, it is advised to start with a balanced diet. It provides us with a good nutritional foundation and can easily be tweaked to meet special dietary needs and health goals.

- **Plant-based diet:**

This diet focuses on plant-based foods such as fruits, vegetables, whole grains, legumes, nuts, and seeds. It is rich in fiber, phytochemicals, and micronutrients. On a plant-based diet you should consume more foods that come from plant sources (McManus, 2018). Animal meat is treated more like a garnish, or a special treat, rather than the centerpiece of a meal.

- **Mediterranean diet:**

This diet emphasizes a diet rich in fruits, vegetables, whole grains, legumes, nuts, and healthy fats, such as olive oil. Moderate amounts of fish, dairy products and poultry is included in this eating plan. Red meat is present in small amounts. This eating plan is considered to be heart-healthy.

- **Low-carb diet:**

This type of diet limits the intake of carbohydrates and focuses on foods high in protein and healthy fats, such as meat, fish, eggs, and nonstarchy vegetables. It can be a restrictive diet and supplementation may be necessary to ensure that our basic nutritional requirements are met. These eating plans are generally used to encourage weight loss. If you decide to follow a low-carb diet, consider the proteins and fats you pick. Limit your intake of meat and high-fat dairy products and other foods high in saturated and trans fats as they may increase the risk of heart disease developing (*Can a low-carb diet help you lose weight?*, 2017).

- **Low-fat diet:**

This type of diet limits the intake of fats and focuses on foods low in fat and high in carbohydrates and proteins, such as fruits, vegetables, whole grains, and lean proteins. Low-fat diets may leave us feeling hungry, and a poorly applied eating plan can encourage deficiencies in fat-soluble vitamins (Olsson, 2022).

- **Specific diets for certain health conditions:**

Some health conditions, such as diabetes, heart disease, and celiac disease, require specific diets, such as a low-sugar, gluten-free, or a low-salt diet.

- **Intermittent fasting:**

In this diet, periods of eating are interspersed with times of fasting. It can involve different methods such as time-restricted eating, alternate-day fasting, or the 5:2 diet (eat normally for five days and fast for two days). It can improve insulin sensitivity and weight loss and positively affect the body's metabolism. While most people can practice intermittent fasting safely, this eating plan is not for everyone. If you're expecting or nursing, skipping meals might not be the greatest method to control your weight. Consult your doctor before beginning an intermittent fasting regimen if you have health issues (Mundi, 2022).

- **Ketogenic diet:**

This type of diet is high in fat, moderate in protein, and very low in carbohydrates, and it helps the body to enter a metabolic state called *ketosis*. In this state our bodies burn fat for energy instead of carbs. It's often used for weight loss and people with certain conditions, such as epilepsy. It should be noted that the ketogenic diet can be very restrictive and that a poorly applied eating plan can have negative health consequences. In many cases we'll need to add quality supplements to a ketogenic diet to ensure that our basic nutritional requirements are met.

- **Paleo diet:**

This type of diet is based on the idea that our ancestors ate similar foods, and it involves eating whole, unprocessed foods. The consumption of fruits, vegetables, meat, fish, and nuts are encouraged. Processed foods, grains, and legumes are not consumed on this eating plan. This eating plan can be a bit restrictive, and supplementation may be necessary to ensure that our basic nutritional requirements are met.

Organic and Gluten-Free Meal Planning

Organic and gluten-free are not considered to be a specific diet meal plan. However, they can be incorporated into different types of diet meal plans. For the sake of clarity, organic and gluten-free meal plans refer to the following:

- **Organic meal planning:** Refers to food that is produced without the use of synthetic pesticides, fertilizers, or genetically modified organisms (GMOs). It is a label that can be applied to certain fruits, vegetables, meats, dairy products, and other foods. Some people eat organic foods because they believe they are healthier or more environmentally friendly.

- **Gluten-free meal planning:** Refers to a diet that eliminates foods containing gluten, a protein found in wheat, barley, and rye. People with celiac disease or nonceliac gluten sensitivity must follow a gluten-free diet to manage their condition. Some people also follow a gluten-free diet because they believe it will improve their health or help them lose weight.

It's possible to follow a diet incorporating organic and gluten-free foods as part of a healthy meal plan, but this would depend on the individual's needs and preferences. It's essential to consult with a healthcare professional, such as a dietitian or nutritionist, to determine if an organic and gluten-free diet is appropriate for you, considering your individual needs, preferences, and health conditions.

Developing a healthy meal plan is to create a structured plan that outlines the types and amounts of foods an individual should eat to meet their nutritional needs and achieve their health goals. It is essential to base the plan on nutrient-dense whole foods, balanced macronutrients, and appropriate portion sizes. A healthy meal plan should be tailored to an individual's unique needs, considering factors such as age, sex, activity level, health status, and dietary restrictions or allergies. It should also take into personal account preferences and cultural food habits. Individuals can improve their overall health and well-being by developing a healthy meal plan, preventing nutrient deficiencies, and achieving specific health goals such as weight loss or managing a medical condition. It can also help an individual to make informed food choices and to monitor their progress.

FOOD DIARY-BASED ACTION

Starting a meal plan can be an overwhelming task, but that's where a food diary makes things a lot easier. By recording what we ate and how it made us feel we'll be able to figure out rather quickly which foods work for the body, and which foods are best avoided. We won't be making any changes to the way the food diary-based activity is completed in this chapter. As you complete your entry, you are encouraged to reflect on the following questions:

- Is my current meal plan working for me? Elaborate on your answer.
- How can I tweak my current eating plan to make it healthier without blowing the budget?
- Do I feel confident about my eating plan? If not, then it is advised to visit a dietician or nutritionist for help.

Meal	How Hungry I Felt (scored from 1-10)	Food Consumed	Amount Consumed	How Satiated I Felt (scored from 1-10)	Did I Eat My Emotions? Why Did I Choose These Foods?
Breakfast	3	Muesli topped with fruit and yogurt.	Had a serving of muesli topped with banana and probiotic yogurt.	7	I'm finding that this breakfast gives me a lot of energy!
Lunch	4	Salad and a fruit smoothie.	Salad with lettuce, tomato, feta cheese, olives, and sweet peppers. Had a blueberry fruit smoothie (prepared at home).	7	Trying to eat a balanced diet with lots of colorful fruits and veggies. I can proudly say I haven't eaten my emotions in a while now!
Dinner	4	Fish and vegetables.	Fried fish with sweet potato chips and spinach (prepared at home).	9	I'm trying to make my favorite takeaway meals healthy.

How Do I Feel About My Body Today? Why?			What Exercise Did I Do Today? How Did I Feel Afterwards?		
I feel completely confident in my skin! I finally feel like my food choices are my own!			*Did 30-minutes of cardio today. It was tiring but I felt great afterwards.*		
Breakfast					
Lunch					
Dinner					
How Do I Feel About My Body Today? Why?			What Exercise Did I Do Today? How Did I Feel Afterwards?		

10

PUTTING YOUR NUTRITION PLAN TOGETHER

P utting together a nutrition plan is vital in achieving your health and wellness goals. A well-rounded nutrition plan should consider your specific needs and goals, as well as your current eating habits and lifestyle. It sounds like a tall order, but can be broken down into three broad steps:

- Determining your daily calorie and baseline nutritional needs.
- From there, you'll need to look at your current eating habits, identifying areas that need improvement.
- Finally, you'll need to make a plan on how to achieve your goals. The plan can include meal

planning, grocery shopping and identifying healthy food options when eating out.

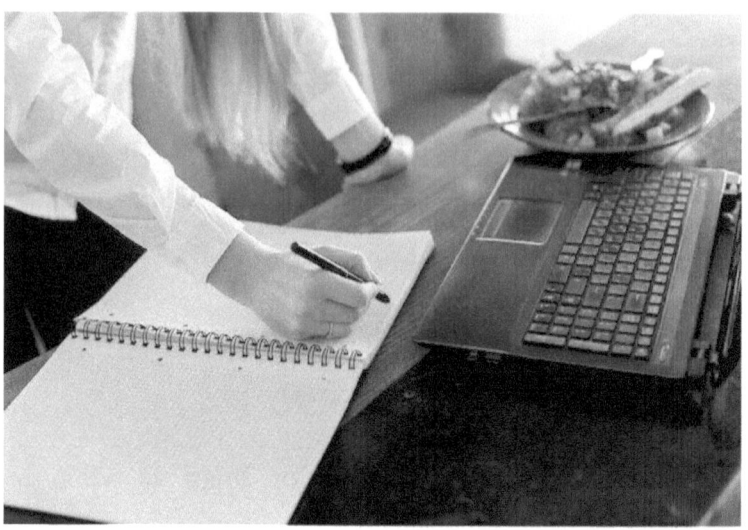

These three broad steps form the foundation of any healthy meal plan. Keep in mind that changes need to be incorporated gradually. This allows the body and taste buds to adjust to the new way of eating. It's also important to monitor your progress and make adjustments as needed. Keep track of your progress by maintaining a food diary, keeping a weight log, or tracking your body measurements. Remember to be consistent and seek support from a registered dietitian or healthcare professional if needed.

The most important thing we need to remember is that a nutrition plan is not a one-time event. Yes, meal planning takes a bit of time and effort, but there is no need (or excuse) to doom yourself to a monotonous diet of roasted fish and steamed greens as Victoria Beckham allegedly did for two and half decades (Ezekiel, 2022). In all honesty, a monotonous diet can be extremely discouraging on a psychological level. There's no denying that we love our food and the flavors that come with it, but if we have the same thing every day we won't look forward to our meals and can become unmotivated to continue with a healthy meal plan.

Change is a constant, so we need to re-evaluate our goals and progress so that we can adjust our eating plan as needed. Most importantly, be kind to yourself! Slip-ups happen. It is a part of life. Slip-ups are not the catastrophic diet-ending, goal-destroying events diet culture have programmed many of us to believe. Life happens, let it be. Enjoy that slice of cake, that oozy brownie, or that hearty holiday meal, but get back on track as soon as possible. Remember, healthy eating is about building on small gains, not punishing ourselves for the occasional slip-up. Now that we've got the basics covered, let's take a closer look at how you can go about to design a healthy meal plan.

BAD INGREDIENTS FOUND IN FOOD

The best piece of advice I can offer is this: Get into the habit of reading food labels. Many potentially harmful ingredients can be found in food. Some examples include:

- **Trans fats:** These unsaturated fats are often used in processed foods to increase shelf life. They have been linked to an increased risk of heart disease. Trans fats were briefly discussed in Chapter 6. Margarines and spreads are common sources of trans fats. Whenever possible, opt for real butter as it does not raise bad cholesterol as much as trans fats do (*Butter vs. margarine: which is healthier?*, n.d.).
- **High fructose corn syrup:** This sweetener is commonly used in processed foods and drinks. It has been linked to obesity and other health problems including fatty liver, insulin resistance, and an increased risk of developing type 2 diabetes (Kubala, 2021).
- **Artificial sweeteners:** These are used to sweeten foods and drinks without adding calories. Some studies have suggested that they may have adverse health effects. If you need something

sweet, rather opt for honey. It has a lower GI value than regular sugar, so it won't spike blood sugar levels so quickly (Armstrong, 2022).

- **Artificial colors:** These are used to enhance food color, but some have been linked to hyperactivity in children and other health issues (Bell, 2017).
- **MSG (monosodium glutamate):** This flavor enhancer is often used in Asian cuisine and processed foods. Even though Uncle Roger (a YouTube personality and comedian) claims it's the "king of flavor" we still need to be wary of this ingredient. Some people may have an allergic reaction to it.
- **Sodium nitrate and nitrite:** This is often used as a preservative and color fixative. Think of that lovely pink color that some cured meats have. That's thanks to sodium nitrate. The organic compound is a known carcinogen (Caballero et al., 2003), so it's not something we should be putting in our bodies.

When we make a habit of checking food labels, we'll be able to make informed dietary choices that can support our health and nutritional goals. Always look for foods that contain more of the nutrients you need and try to avoid the bad ingredients listed above as much as possible.

HEALTHY CHOICE EATING

This point can't be stressed enough: Eating a healthy diet is important to maintaining overall health and well-being. Fortunately, there are many different ways to make healthy food choices! Some general guidelines include the following:

- **Eating a variety of nutrient-dense foods:** This includes fruits and vegetables, whole grains, lean protein, and healthy fats. These foods provide essential nutrients such as vitamins, minerals, and fiber.
- **Limiting processed and high-calorie foods:** Processed foods often contain added sugars, sodium, and unhealthy fats, which can contribute to weight gain and other health problems.
- **Watch the portion size:** Overeating any food can lead to weight gain, and it's important to be aware of how much we consume. Portion size can be tricky to come to grips with at first. If you find yourself overeating, try to use smaller plates and measure your food using measuring

cups. Try not to pick at leftovers and give yourself 20 minutes before going for a second helping (*Top tips for portion control*, 2018). These small adjustments (especially the 20-minute wait time) will go a long way to helping you master portion control in a healthy way.

- **Eating regularly:** Eating smaller, more frequent meals throughout the day can help control hunger and prevent overeating.

- **Staying hydrated:** Drinking water and other noncaloric beverages can help keep you hydrated and full. We often mistake thirst for hunger, so it is a good idea to reach for a glass of water before having a meal. If you're still hungry after drinking water or other non-caloric beverages, then you should eat.

- **Eating mindfully:** Paying attention to what you are eating and savoring the flavors and textures of your food can help you enjoy your meals more and eat less. Take the time to savor and enjoy your food, rather than eating on the go or in front of the TV. You'll be surprised at the difference this simple adjustment makes!

- **Planning ahead:** Planning meals and snacks in advance can help you make healthier choices and avoid last-minute decisions that may lead to unhealthy options.

These simple guidelines can be applied to any meal plan. When practiced consistently it will pay dividends in the long run and can help us reach health and weight loss goals. Try to apply these guidelines even when you find yourself slipping up, especially mindful eating. By doing so, your progress won't be derailed as badly as you feared.

ADOPT A HEALTHY WAY OF THINKING INSTEAD OF DIETING

Adopting a healthy way of thinking about food involves shifting your focus from restrictive dieting and weight loss to nourishing your body with nutrient-dense foods. It has to do with listening to your body's hunger and fullness cues. In other words, adopting a new meal plan should be viewed as a lifestyle change. Here are some ways to help you adopt a healthy way of thinking about food:

- **Ditch the diet mentality:**

Diets often have a start and end date and focus on weight loss. Instead, focus on adopting healthy habits that you can maintain long-term. Tell yourself that you are not on a diet but have adopted a healthy way of eating instead. Improving your relationship with food should take precedence over weight loss goals. Weight loss tends to come naturally when we have a healthy relationship with food and listen to our bodies.

- **Listen to your body:**

Learn to recognize and respond to your body's signals of hunger and fullness. Eating when you're hungry and stopping when you're full can help prevent overeating.

- **Diversify your food choices:**

Eating various nutrient-dense foods can help you get all the essential nutrients your body needs. Also, it adds variety to our meal plan, preventing us from becoming bored with the same dishes. Don't be afraid to experiment and try new foods. You might discover a new favorite in the process!

- **Don't restrict certain foods:**

Restricting certain foods can lead to cravings and overeating. Instead, allow yourself to enjoy all foods in moderation. The operative word here is moderation. Yes, you can have that chocolate ganache cake you've been craving! Rather than having a big, fat slice of cake, opt for a thin slice. This will help to limit the calories you are adding, while satisfying that sweet tooth. It's not recommended to indulge in sweet things too often, but once in a while won't derail things either. The only time when we really should restrict foods are when we are placed on a special meal plan by a medical professional due to health concerns.

- **Embrace the pleasure of eating:**

Food is not only for nourishment but also for pleasure and enjoyment, enjoy it! There's a world of flavor to explore and tons of memorable food moments that is simply waiting to be discovered.

- **Be kind to yourself:**

Healthy eating is a journey of self-discovery. On that journey we'll have many interesting adventures and some misadventures, so don't be hard on yourself when you slip up. Everyone slips up from time to time. It is natural and human to do so. You deserve to feel wonderful, so embrace the journey with a good measure of kindness and compassion towards yourself.

- **Focus on health, not weight:**

Health is not a number on a scale. It's about how you feel and function.

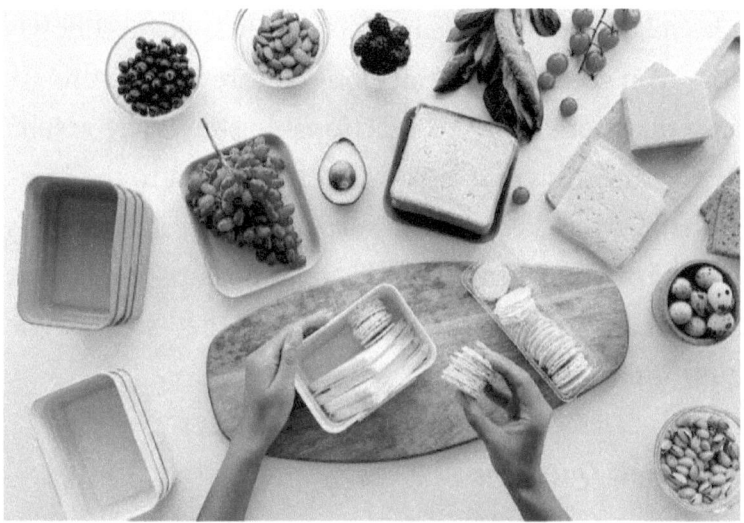

Remember that healthy eating is not about perfection but about making better choices most of the time and learning to listen to and trust your body. It is important to remember that everyone's body is different, and there is no one-size-fits-all approach to healthy eating. So, it is imperative that you find a way of eating that works for you and your lifestyle and focus on overall health and well-being rather than solely on weight loss. By implementing the steps outlined below, you can achieve your nutrition and weight management goals successfully. Follow these steps closely and it will save you years of frustration!

THE PLAN THAT WORKS FOR YOU

This plan couldn't be simpler! It takes all the knowledge you've gained in this book and refines it into six easy questions and seven actionable steps. The result? A way of eating that is completely tailored to the individual! I won't keep you in suspense any longer, so let's kickstart your healthy food relationship. Be honest and realistic when you answer the six simple questions.

Six Simple Questions

- **What are my specific nutritional needs?** These may include calorie and macronutrient requirements and recommended daily intake for vitamins and minerals.
- **How much do I need to eat?** Your daily calorie needs will depend on age, sex, weight, and activity level. It's important to determine your daily calorie needs so that you can plan your meals and snacks accordingly.
- **What are my health goals?** Are you looking to lose weight, improve athletic performance,

manage a medical condition, or improve overall health?

- **What are my current eating habits?** This includes the types of foods you eat and when and how you eat them.
- **What are my food preferences and restrictions?** This includes allergies, food intolerances, cultural or religious restrictions, and personal preferences.
- **What is my lifestyle like?** Your work schedule, level of physical activity, and access to healthy food options can all affect your ability to follow a nutrition plan.

The answers to these questions will help lay a solid foundation for your personalized nutrition plan. Take your time and reflect on the answers carefully. When you are ready, proceed to the next part outlined below.

Seven Step Plan to Get Your Nutrition Plan Initiated

Now that you have the foundation for your nutrition plan, you'll need to take a series of steps to truly get the ball rolling.

- **Dietary Action One: Identify Nutritional goals:** Identify the changes you want to make to your diet, and set measurable and achievable goals. This could be increasing your fruit and vegetable intake, reducing your added sugar intake, or increasing your protein intake.

- **Dietary Action Two: Initiate the plan:** Once you have identified your goals, make a plan on how you are going to achieve them. This can include meal planning, grocery shopping, and identifying healthy food options when eating out.

- **Dietary Action Three: Implement changes gradually:** Changing your diet overnight can be overwhelming. Instead, implement changes gradually, allowing your body and taste buds to adjust.

- **Dietary Action Four: Track your progress:** Keep track of your progress by maintaining a food diary, keeping a weight log, or tracking your body measurements.

- **Dietary Action Five: Be consistent:** Consistency is key when trying to make a change, so stick to your plan as much as possible. Remember that it is okay to slip up and make mistakes. Just get back on track as soon as possible.

- **Dietary Action Six: Re-evaluate and adjust:** As you progress, re-evaluate your goals and progress, and adjust your plan as needed. A nutrition plan should not be a one-time event. It should be a continuous process.

- **Dietary Action Seven: Get additional support:** Consider working with a registered dietitian or healthcare professional to help create a safe and tailored plan for your specific needs.

The best part of this plan is that it puts the power of making informed food choices back in your hands. Remember that changing your diet takes time and effort, be patient with yourself, and celebrate small wins along the way. Answering these questions will help create a comprehensive and personalized nutrition plan that considers your specific needs, goals, and lifestyle. Working with a registered dietitian or healthcare professional is important to ensure that your plan is safe and appropriate.

SEVEN-STEP ACTION PLAN IN PRACTICE

Implementing the seven-step action plan could not be easier. Start by laying the foundation by answering the *Six Simple Questions*. From there, we can make meaningful changes to the way we eat by applying the seven dietary action steps.

- **Define your health goals:** Start by identifying your health goals. Whether it be losing weight, improving your digestion, reducing your risk of chronic disease or gaining mass, it is important to know the direction you want to go so you can plan accordingly.

- **Assess current habits**: Take a close look at your current habits and routines. How are they helping or harming your health goals? This should include eating patterns, exercise routines and stress management.

- **Spot potential obstacles:** What challenges may arise as you work towards your health goals? This could be a busy work schedule, lack of time, low motivation, financial constraints and obstacles that can make attaining your goals difficult.

- **Create the plan:** Now that you've laid the groundwork by defining health goals, assessing current habits and spotting obstacles, you'll need to create a step-by-step plan that will help you achieve your health goals. Include specific actions such as meal planning, scheduling workouts or making time for a stress-relieving activity that you enjoy.

- **Monitor progress:** Now that all the hard prep work is done, keep track of your progress through a food diary or fitness tracker. You'll need to stay accountable and make adjustments to your plan as needed. Consistency is key.

- **Stay motivated:** Most eating plans fail because we lose motivation. By setting achievable goals and rewarding yourself for progress, we can stay motivated for longer. An accountability partner and supportive community can be great sources of motivation as well.

- **Evaluate and adjust the plan:** Change is a constant in our lives so our plan will need adjustment from time to time. Regularly evaluate your progress and adjust the plan as needed. It is important to remain flexible and willing to adapt to changes in our lives (such as a new job or family situation).

The seven action steps mentioned above will help you create a clear and actionable plan to achieve your health goals and can improve your overall well-being. Don't forget to revisit your plan from time to time and adjust it as needed. Most importantly, remember to be kind to yourself. Meaningful change can take time, but you already took the first big step towards achieving your health goals!

READY TO HELP LIGHT THE PATH FOR OTHERS?

No matter where we are on our nutritional journey, we all need guidance… and you're in the perfect position to offer it.

Simply by leaving your honest opinion of this book on Amazon, you can help other people understand that the nutritional regime that works best for them is one that takes 7 key factors into account.

WANT TO HELP OTHERS?

I'm so grateful for your support… and I just know thousands of other readers will be too. A healthy meal plan can make us feel on top of the world… and nothing beats helping others feel exactly the same way!

CONCLUSION

What a journey of discovery we've been on! We discovered the factors that influence our food choices. From the cultural and social influences to the impact of the food industry, we have learned that what we eat is shaped by more than just our taste buds. We have also learned about the negative impact of diet culture on our relationship with food. By understanding the role of biochemistry in nutrition, we have gone back to the basics and discovered that fat is not the enemy, and not all carbs are created equal. We have also learned about the risks associated with consuming too much or too little of any nutrient.

It is common for mainstream weight loss gurus to focus on a number on the scale as a measure of health, but we now know that achieving a healthy body composition is more important. With the knowledge and tools gained from this powerful food education, you can take control of your food choices and make meaningful changes to the way you eat. By following our seven-step plan, you can develop a healthy relationship with food, which will help you achieve the healthy body you've always desired.

Remember, a healthy relationship with food starts with knowing your worth and loving yourself, including your flaws. Self-care is not selfish, and everyone deserves to feel their best. Achieving your goals will require effort, but it is all achievable when we embrace the power of small steps. Every day counts, and the transformation is about who we become in the process.

Now that you have all the tools to develop a healthy relationship with food, we encourage you to go out there and enjoy a wonderful food adventure! If this book has helped you in any way, please leave a review where you purchased this book. By doing so, you'll be helping others discover a way of eating that works for them too!

I also invite you to visit my website, F4URY.com, where you can connect with me. I believe that everyone has a unique journey, and I would love to hear about yours. On my website, you'll find a wealth of resources to help you discover new ways to find meaning in life, including information on topics I'm passionate about, such as health, love, wealth, and happiness. Whether you're looking to improve your own life or make a positive impact on the world around you, F4URY.com is the perfect place to start your journey toward a brighter future.

EXPLORE MORE OF THE AUTHOR'S WORK THAT COMPLEMENTS THIS BOOK

Unlock your potential for success with "Knowing What You Think About Is Where You Will Go". This life-changing book provides proven strategies and tools to help you take control of your success and turn your dreams into a reality. Don't let limiting beliefs and negative mindsets hold you back any longer - grab your copy today and start transforming your life.

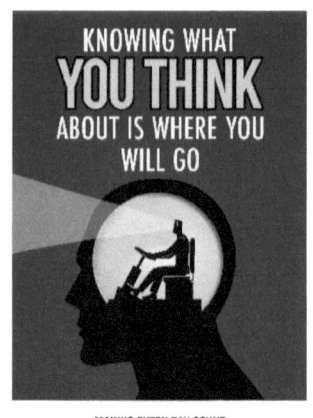

If you enjoyed this book you can purchase this book where you originally purchased this one. Thank you for your support!

REFERENCES

REFERENCES

Access to foods that support healthy dietary patterns. (n.d.). U.S. Department of Health and Human Services. https://health.gov/healthypeople/priority-areas/social-determinants-health/literature-summaries/access-foods-support-healthy-dietary-patterns

Anaphylaxis - symptoms and causes. (2021, October 2). Mayo Clinic. https://www.mayoclinic.org/diseases-conditions/anaphylaxis/symptoms-causes/syc-20351468

Anderson, C. (2021, April 6). *A guy drank 2 liters of fiber supplement to cleanse his insides and nearly died because of it.* BroBible. https://brobible.com/culture/article/guy-drank-much-fiber-supplement-disaster-story/

Appelhans, B. M., Milliron, B.-J., Woolf, K., Johnson, T. J., Pagoto, S. L., Schneider, K. L., Whited, M. C., & Ventrelle, J. C. (2012). Socioeconomic Status, Energy Cost, and Nutrient Content of Supermarket Food Purchases. *American Journal of Preventive Medicine, 42*(4), 398–402. https://doi.org/10.1016/j.amepre.2011.12.007

ARFID. (n.d.). Beat Eating Disorders. https://www.beateatingdisorders.org.uk/get-information-and-support/about-eating-disorders/types/arfid/

Armstrong, L. (2022, January 9). *Is honey better than sugar? A dietitian shares why she loves its health benefits—and her favorite ways to use it.* CNBC. https://www.cnbc.com/2022/01/09/is-honey-better-than-sugar-a-dietitian-shares-why-she-loves-its-health-benefits.html

Babatunde-Sowole, O. O., Power, T., Davidson, P., Ballard, C., & Jackson, D. (2018). Exploring the diet and lifestyle changes contributing to weight gain among Australian West African women following migration: A qualitative study. *Contemporary Nurse, 54*(2), 150–159. https://doi.org/10.1080/10376178.2018.1459760

Barclay, K. J., Edling, C., & Rydgren, J. (2013). Peer clustering of exercise and eating behaviors among young adults in Sweden: a cross-sectional study of egocentric network data. *BMC Public Health, 13*(1). https://doi.org/10.1186/1471-2458-13-784

Beal, T., & Ortenzi, F. (2022). Priority Micronutrient Density in Foods. *Frontiers in Nutrition, 9.* https://doi.org/10.3389/fnut.2022.806566

Bell, B. (2017, January 7). *Food Dyes: Harmless or Harmful?* Healthline; healthline. https://www.healthline.com/nutrition/food-dyes

Biotin. (n.d.). National Institutes of Health. https://ods.od.nih.gov/fact sheets/Biotin-HealthProfessional/

Body fat testing through underwater weighing. (n.d.). MyNetDiary. https://www.mynetdiary.com/body-fat-testing-through-underwater-weighing.html

Body image and diets. (2013). Better Health Channel. https://www.better health.vic.gov.au/health/healthyliving/body-image-and-diets

Boothby, E. J., Clark, M. S., & Bargh, J. A. (2014). Shared Experiences Are Amplified. *Psychological Science, 25*(12), 2209–2216. https://doi.org/10.1177/0956797614551162

Brown, Z., & Tiggemann, M. (2021). Celebrity influence on body image and eating disorders: A review. *Journal of Health Psychology, 27*(5), 135910532098831. https://doi.org/10.1177/1359105320988312

Burns, R. D., Fu, Y., & Constantino, N. (2019). Measurement agreement in percent body fat estimates among laboratory and field assessments in college students: Use of equivalence testing. *PLOS ONE, 14*(3), e0214029. https://doi.org/10.1371/journal.pone.0214029

Butter vs. margarine: which is healthier? (n.d.). Healthline. https://www.healthline.com/nutrition/butter-vs-margarine

Caballero, B., Trugo, L. C., & Finglas, P. M. (2003). *Encyclopedia of food sciences and nutrition / Vol. 9, [Soy-V].* Academic Press, Cop.

Canker sore - symptoms and causes. (n.d.). Mayo Clinic. https://www.mayoclinic.org/diseases-conditions/canker-sore/symptoms-causes/syc-20370615

Can a low-carb diet help you lose weight? (2017). Mayo Clinic. https://

www.mayoclinic.org/healthy-lifestyle/weight-loss/in-depth/low-carb-diet/art-20045831

Carbohydrates: How carbs fit into a healthy diet. (2022). Mayo Clinic. https://www.mayoclinic.org/healthy-lifestyle/nutrition-and-healthy-eating/in-depth/carbohydrates/art-20045705

Carreiro, A. L., Dhillon, J., Gordon, S., Higgins, K. A., Jacobs, A. G., McArthur, B. M., Redan, B. W., Rivera, R. L., Schmidt, L. R., & Mattes, R. D. (2016). The Macronutrients, Appetite, and Energy Intake. *Annual Review of Nutrition, 36*(1), 73–103. https://doi.org/10.1146/annurev-nutr-121415-112624

Carson, L. (2019, July 11). *Body composition vs BMI, what's the difference?* Hyatt Training. https://hyatttraining.com/body-composition-vs-bmi/

Cavazza, N., Graziani, A. R., & Guidetti, M. (2011). Looking for the "right" amount to eat at the restaurant: Social influence effects when ordering. *Social Influence, 6*(4), 274–290. https://doi.org/10.1080/15534510.2011.632130

Childhood obesity facts. (2022, May 17). CDC. https://www.cdc.gov/obesity/data/childhood.html

Chung, S.-Y., Butts, C. L., Maleki, S. J., & Champagne, E. T. (2003). Linking Peanut Allergenicity to the Processes of Maturation, Curing, and Roasting. *Journal of Agricultural and Food Chemistry, 51*(15), 4273–4277. https://doi.org/10.1021/jf021212d

Cirino, E. (2019, January 9). *Detox tea: side effects, purported benefits, and how they work.* Healthline. https://www.healthline.com/health/detox-tea-side-effects

Daryanani, A. (2021, January 28). *"Diet culture" & social media.* Recreation.ucsd.edu. https://recreation.ucsd.edu/2021/01/diet-culture-social-media/

David, E. (2020, February 28). *Teens "especially vulnerable" to junk food advertising, experts say.* ABC News. https://abcnews.go.com/Health/teens-vulnerable-junk-food-advertising-experts/story?id=69060220

Diet culture throughout history. (2022, September 13). Embody Health London. https://embodyhealthlondon.com/diet-culture-through

out-history/

Dieter, B. (n.d.). *The science of energy balance: How it Factors Into Metabolism.* NASM. https://blog.nasm.org/a-guide-to-energy-balance

Does metabolism matter in weight loss? (2015, July 16). Harvard Health; Harvard Health. https://www.health.harvard.edu/diet-and-weight-loss/does-metabolism-matter-in-weight-loss

Dvorak, A. (2021, November 5). *Top 13 high thermic effect foods to boost your metabolism.* Fitbod. https://fitbod.me/blog/high-thermic-effect-foods/

Dysgeusia. (n.d.). Midwest Ear, Nose And Throat. https://www.midwest ent.com/dysgeusia#:~:text=Vitamin%20or%20mineral%20deficien cies%E2%80%94Deficiencies

Earnesty, D. (2018). *Do food cues really have an influence on our food intake?* Nutrition. https://www.canr.msu.edu/news/ do_food_cues_really_have_an_influence_on_our_food_intake

Ezekiel, L. (2022, September 3). *I tried Victoria Beckham's super-strict diet - how can anyone live like this?* The Sun. https://www.thesun.co.uk/ fabulous/food/19660808/victoria-beckham-super-strict-diet/

Ezzeldin, H. (2022, September 19). *8 micronutrients important for meta-bolic health.* HealthifyMe. https://www.healthifyme.com/blog/ micronutrients-for-metabolic-health/

Fact sheet: an adjustment to global poverty lines. (n.d.). World Bank. https://www.worldbank.org/en/news/factsheet/2022/05/02/fact-sheet-an-adjustment-to-global-poverty-lines

Facts and statistics. (n.d.). Food Allergy Research and Education (FARE). https://www.foodallergy.org/resources/facts-and-statistics

Fat hydrogenation. (2021, May 27). Wikipedia. https://en.wikipedia.org/ wiki/Fat_hydrogenation

Fat: the facts. (2022, February 23). NHS. https://www.nhs.uk/live-well/ eat-well/food-types/different-fats-nutrition/

Fearnow, B. (2017, May 6). *Study: Rich people love eating fast food as much as everyone else.* Study Finds. https://studyfinds.org/fast-food-rich-poor-study/

Fiber. (2012, September 18). Harvard T.H. Chan. https://www.hsph.

harvard.edu/nutritionsource/carbohydrates/fiber/

Florida man only eats mac and cheese for last 17 years. (2023, January 6). *ESPN Southwest Florida*. https://espnswfl.com/2023/01/06/flor ida-man-only-eats-mac-and-cheese-for-last-17-years/

Food allergies and fatigue. (n.d.). Moss Center Integrative Medicine. https://mosscenterforintegrativemedicine.com/treatments/ fatigue/food-allergies-fatigue

Food allergy versus food intolerance. (n.d.). Allergy Insider. https://www. thermofisher.com/allergy/za/en/living-with-allergies/food-aller gies/food-allergy-vs-food-intolerance.html?

Food insecurity. (n.d.). U.S. Department of Health and Human Services. https://health.gov/healthypeople/priority-areas/social-determi nants-health/literature-summaries/food-insecurity

Food prices for nutrition datahub: global statistics on the cost and affordability of healthy diets. (n.d.). World Bank. https://www.worldbank.org/en/ programs/icp/brief/foodpricesfornutrition

Fothergill, E., Guo, J., Howard, L., Kerns, J. C., Knuth, N. D., Brychta, R., Chen, K. Y., Skarulis, M. C., Walter, M., Walter, P. J., & Hall, K. D. (2016). Persistent metabolic adaptation 6 years after "The Biggest Loser" competition. *Obesity (Silver Spring, Md.), 24*(8), 1612–1619. https://doi.org/10.1002/oby.21538

Freeman, K. (n.d.). *Organisation and meal planning for busy people.* The Healthy Eating Hub. https://healthyeatinghub.com.au/meal-plan ning-for-busy-people/

Garrick, N. (2017, March 9). *Healthy muscles matter.* National Institute of Arthritis and Musculoskeletal and Skin Diseases. https://www. niams.nih.gov/health-topics/kids/healthy-muscles

Griffin, R. (2022, March 29). *Don't dismiss the data: why baseline tests are essential to achieving optimal health - griffin concierge medical.* Griffin Concierge Medical. https://griffinconciergemedical.com/baseline-tests-are-essential-to-achieving-optimal-health/

Guest, E. (2016). Photo editing: enhancing social media images to reflect appearance ideals. *Journal of Aesthetic Nursing, 5*(9), 444–446. https://doi.org/10.12968/joan.2016.5.9.444

Gunnars, K. (2018). *22 high-fiber foods you should eat.* Healthline. https://

www.healthline.com/nutrition/22-high-fiber-foods

Gut health: why is it important? (2022). Franciscan Health. https://www.franciscanhealth.org/community/blog/gut-health-why-is-it-important

Hadley, C. (2006). Food allergies on the rise? Determining the prevalence of food allergies, and how quickly it is increasing, is the first step in tackling the problem. *EMBO Reports, 7*(11), 1080–1083. https://doi.org/10.1038/sj.embor.7400846

Handbury, J., Rahkovsky, I., & Schnell, M. (2015). What drives nutritional disparities?: retail access and food purchases across the socioeconomic spectrum. *National Bureau of Economic Research.*

Hawkins, L. K., Farrow, C., & Thomas, J. M. (2020). Do perceived norms of social media users' eating habits and preferences predict our own food consumption and BMI? *Appetite, 149,* 104611. https://doi.org/10.1016/j.appet.2020.104611

Heavner, B. (2019). *How does texture affect taste?* Charlotte Eye Ear Nose and Throat Associates. https://www.ceenta.com/news-blog/how-texture-affects-taste

Heger, E. (2022, May 19). *The sneaky ways social media can sabotage your body image — and 3 easy tips to help you break the cycle.* Insider. https://www.insider.com/guides/health/mental-health/how-social-media-affects-body-image

Henderson, E. (2022, June 14). *Taste-related genes may play a role in determining food choices, finds study.* News-Medical.net. https://www.news-medical.net/news/20220614/Taste-related-genes-may-play-a-role-in-determining-food-choices-finds-study.aspx

Hermans, R. C. J., Larsen, J. K., Lochbuehler, K., Nederkoorn, C., Herman, C. P., & Engels, R. C. M. E. (2012). The power of social influence over food intake: examining the effects of attentional bias and impulsivity. *British Journal of Nutrition, 109*(3), 572–580. https://doi.org/10.1017/s0007114512001390

Higgs, S., & Thomas, J. (2016). Social influences on eating. *Current Opinion in Behavioral Sciences, 9*(9), 1–6. https://doi.org/10.1016/j.cobeha.2015.10.005

How can advertisements influence your food choices? (2020, January 22).

Center for Nutrition in Schools (CNS). https://cns.ucdavis.edu/ news/how-can-advertisements-influence-your-food-choices

Hui, S. (2022). *What is healthism? ideas, examples, and how to confront it.* GoodRx. https://www.goodrx.com/healthcare-access/patient-advo cacy/what-is-healthism

Institute of Medicine. (2000). *Dietary reference intakes for vitamin c, vitamin e, selenium, and carotenoids.* National Academies Press. https://doi.org/10.17226/9810

Is a food allergy causing you inflammation? (2018, February 21). Mile High Spine and Pain Center. https://milehighspine.com/is-a-food-allergy-causing-you-inflammation/

Kana"An, H., Saadeh, R., Zruqait, A., & Alenezi, M. (2021). Knowledge, attitude, and practice of healthy eating among public school teachers in Kuwait. *Journal of Public Health Research.* https://doi.org/ 10.4081/jphr.2021.2223

Kawafune, K., Hachiya, T., Nogawa, S., Takahashi, S., Jia, H., Saito, K., & Kato, H. (2020). Strong association between the 12q24 locus and sweet taste preference in the Japanese population revealed by genome-wide meta-analysis. *Journal of Human Genetics, 65*(11), 939–947. https://doi.org/10.1038/s10038-020-0787-x

Kessler, K., & Pivovarova-Ramich, O. (2019). Meal timing, aging, and metabolic health. *International Journal of Molecular Sciences, 20*(8), 1911. https://doi.org/10.3390/ijms20081911

Khan Mirajkar, K. (2021). *Bioavailability of nutrients – definition and importance.* Nutrova. https://nutrova.com/blogs/health/bioavailabil ity-of-nutrients-definition-importance

Klucharev, V., Hytönen, K., Rijpkema, M., Smidts, A., & Fernández, G. (2009). Reinforcement Learning Signal Predicts Social Conformity. *Neuron, 61*(1), 140–151. https://doi.org/10.1016/j.neuron.2008. 11.027

Kolata, G. (2007, July 25). Obesity spreads to friends, study concludes. *The New York Times.* https://www.nytimes.com/2007/07/25/ health/25iht-fat.4.6830240.html

Kubala, J. (2021, August 30). *12 common foods with high fructose corn syrup.* Healthline. https://www.healthline.com/nutrition/foods-with-high-fructose-corn-syrup

Landes, E. (2022, January 26). *9 hormones that affect weight — and how to improve them.* Healthline. https://www.healthline.com/nutrition/9-fixes-for-weight-hormones#1.-Insulin

Larger portion sizes contribute to U.S. obesity problem. (2013). National Heart, Lung, and Blood Institute. https://www.nhlbi.nih.gov/health/educational/wecan/news-events/matte1.htm

Lee, S. Y., & Gallagher, D. (2008). Assessment methods in human body composition. *Current Opinion in Clinical Nutrition and Metabolic Care, 11*(5), 566–572. https://doi.org/10.1097/mco.0b013e32830b5f23

Lowry, D. W., & Tomiyama, A. J. (2015). Air displacement plethysmography versus dual-energy x-ray absorptiometry in underweight, normal-weight, and overweight/obese individuals. *PLOS ONE, 10*(1), e0115086. https://doi.org/10.1371/journal.pone.0115086

Mahtani, P. (2020). *Struggling with food sensitivities? Your hormones may be playing a role.* Pollie. https://www.pollie.co/blog/food-sensitivities-hormones

Marcin, A. (2018, August 28). *Emotional eating: what you should know.* Healthline; Healthline Media. https://www.healthline.com/health/emotional-eating

Marvin, K. (2022, December 1). *Health and nutrition.* The Dream Center. https://www.thedreamcenterfw.com/post/women-over-take-men-in-college-degrees

Masrul, M., & Nindrea, R. D. (2019). Dietary fibre protective against colorectal cancer patients in Asia: a meta-analysis. *Open Access Macedonian Journal of Medical Sciences, 7*(10), 1723–1727. https://doi.org/10.3889/oamjms.2019.265

Mather, K. (2023, January 5). "Toxic" fitness influencer reveals common tactics used to trick followers for engagement: "You probably don't know about [this]." *Yahoo News.* https://www.yahoo.com/news/toxic-fitness-influencer-reveals-common-tactics-used-to-trick-followers-for-engagement-you-probably-dont-know-about-this-164912708.html?guccounter=1&guce_referrer=

McManus, K. D. (2018, September 26). *What is a plant-based diet and*

why should you try it? Harvard Health. https://www.health.harvard.
edu/blog/what-is-a-plant-based-diet-and-why-should-you-try-it-
2018092614760

Metabolism. (2012). Better Health Channel. https://www.betterhealth.
vic.gov.au/health/conditionsandtreatments/metabolism

Mikstas, C. (2021). *How other senses affect what you eat.* WebMD. https://
www.webmd.com/diet/ss/slideshow-other-senses-affect-eating

Miller, J. L. (2013). Iron deficiency anemia: a common and curable
disease. *Cold Spring Harbor Perspectives in Medicine, 3*(7). https://doi.
org/10.1101/cshperspect.a011866

Moller, J. (2021). *What should I eat? Who to blame for your bad eating
habits?* BioCertica. https://biocertica.com/blogs/nutrition-well-
being/food-preferences-who-to-blame-for-my-sweet-tooth

Monsivais, P., Aggarwal, A., & Drewnowski, A. (2010). Are socio-
economic disparities in diet quality explained by diet cost? *Journal
of Epidemiology and Community Health, 66*(6), 530–535. https://doi.
org/10.1136/jech.2010.122333

Moore, B. (2021, November 1). *How to use skinfold calipers to measure
body fat percentage.* Legion Athletics. https://legionathletics.com/
body-fat-calipers/

Muhlheim, L. (2017, August 30). *Body image and eating disorders.*
Verywell Mind. https://www.verywellmind.com/body-image-and-
eating-disorders-4149424

Mundi, M. (2022, May 5). *Is intermittent fasting good for you?* Mayo
Clinic. https://www.mayoclinic.org/healthy-lifestyle/nutrition-
and-healthy-eating/expert-answers/intermittent-fasting/faq-
20441303

Neeland, I. J., Turer, A. T., Ayers, C. R., Berry, J. D., Rohatgi, A., Das, S.
R., Khera, A., Vega, G. L., McGuire, D. K., Grundy, S. M., & de
Lemos, J. A. (2015). Body fat distribution and incident cardiovas-
cular disease in obese adults. *Journal of the American College of
Cardiology, 65*(19), 2150–2151. https://doi.org/10.1016/j.jacc.2015.
01.061

Nutrient-dense food. (2011). National Cancer Institute; Cancer.gov.

https://www.cancer.gov/publications/dictionaries/cancer-terms/def/nutrient-dense-food

Obesity. (2019). NHS; NHS. https://www.nhs.uk/conditions/obesity/causes/

Olsson, R. (2022). *Pros and cons of a low-fat diet and is it for you?* Banner Health. https://www.bannerhealth.com/healthcareblog/teach-me/low-fat-diet

Pechey, R., & Monsivais, P. (2016). Socioeconomic inequalities in the healthiness of food choices: Exploring the contributions of food expenditures. *Preventive Medicine, 88,* 203–209. https://doi.org/10.1016/j.ypmed.2016.04.012

Pechey, R., Monsivais, P., Ng, Y.-L., & Marteau, T. M. (2015). Why don't poor men eat fruit? Socioeconomic differences in motivations for fruit consumption. *Appetite, 84,* 271–279. https://doi.org/10.1016/j.appet.2014.10.022

Peter Herman, C., Polivy, J., Pliner, P., & Vartanian, L. R. (2015). Mechanisms underlying the portion-size effect. *Physiology & Behavior, 144,* 129–136. https://doi.org/10.1016/j.physbeh.2015.03.025

Petre, A. (2019, November 4). *8 common signs of vitamin deficiency, plus how to fix them.* Healthline. https://www.healthline.com/nutrition/vitamin-deficiency

Picco, M. F. (n.d.). *Should you take daily fiber supplements?* Mayo Clinic. https://www.mayoclinic.org/healthy-lifestyle/nutrition-and-healthy-eating/expert-answers/fiber-supplements/faq-20058513

Piqueras-Fiszman, B., Harrar, V., Alcaide, J., & Spence, C. (2011). Does the weight of the dish influence our perception of food? *Food Quality and Preference, 22*(8), 753–756. https://doi.org/10.1016/j.foodqual.2011.05.009

Pope, A. (2021). *Mind over matter? Recognizing your hunger cues.* UAB News. https://www.uab.edu/news/youcanuse/item/12248-mind-over-matter-recognizing-your-hunger-cues

Poteet, M. (2021, May 6). *Dangerous diet pills you should avoid | weight loss pills.* The Compounding Pharmacy of America. https://compoundingrxusa.com/blog/dangerous-diet-pills-avoid/

Prinsen, S., de Ridder, D. T. D., & de Vet, E. (2013). Eating by example. Effects of environmental cues on dietary decisions. *Appetite, 70*, 1–5. https://doi.org/10.1016/j.appet.2013.05.023

Puri, A. (2021, November 2). *Does dehydration affect one's metabolism?* Ultrahuman Healthcare. https://ultrahuman.com/blog/does-dehy dration-affect-metabolism/

Ransom, W. (2017, December 6). *The difference between authentic Japanese sushi and sushi around the world.* The Sushi FAQ. https:// www.sushifaq.com/sushiotaku/2013/11/15/difference-authentic-japanese-sushi-sushi-around-world/

Ratini, M. (2021, June 2). *What is body composition?* WebMD. https:// www.webmd.com/fitness-exercise/what-is-body-composition

Red meat and colon cancer. (2008, January 1). Harvard Health Publishing. https://www.health.harvard.edu/staying-healthy/red-meat-and-colon-cancer

Reichelt, A. (2019, November 14). *Your brain on sugar: What the science actually says.* The Conversation. https://theconversation.com/your-brain-on-sugar-what-the-science-actually-says-126581

Reilly, C. (n.d.). *Top 20 foods high in antioxidants.* https://www.stjohns. health/documents/content/top-20-foods-high-in-antioxidants.pdf

Robinson, E., Tobias, T., Shaw, L., Freeman, E., & Higgs, S. (2011). Social matching of food intake and the need for social acceptance. *Appetite, 56*(3), 747–752. https://doi.org/10.1016/j.appet.2011. 03.001

Roser, M., & Ritchie, H. (2013). Hunger and undernourishment. *Our World in Data.* https://ourworldindata.org/hunger-and-undernour ishment#moderate-food-insecurity

Ruddock, H. K., Brunstrom, J. M., Vartanian, L. R., & Higgs, S. (2019). A systematic review and meta-analysis of the social facilitation of eating. *The American Journal of Clinical Nutrition, 110*(4), 842–861. https://doi.org/10.1093/ajcn/nqz155

Salmon, S. J., Fennis, B. M., de Ridder, D. T. D., Adriaanse, M. A., & de Vet, E. (2014). Health on impulse: When low self-control promotes healthy food choices. *Health Psychology, 33*(2), 103–109. https://doi. org/10.1037/a0031785

Satrazemis, E. (2021, March 23). *What is body composition? and 5 ways to measure it.* Www.trifectanutrition.com. https://www.trifectanutrition.com/blog/what-is-body-composition-and-how-to-measure-it

Sawhney, V. (2021, August 6). *Weirdly true: we are what we eat.* Harvard Business Review. https://hbr.org/2021/08/weirdly-true-we-are-what-we-eat

Serotonin. (2022, March 18). Cleveland Clinic. https://my.clevelandclinic.org/health/articles/22572-serotonin

Sheth, V. R. (2023). *How can my emotional state affect my eating habits? | Emotional Eating.* Sharecare. https://www.sharecare.com/health/emotional-eating/how-emotional-state-affect-eating

Singla, P. (2010). Metabolic effects of obesity: A review. *World Journal of Diabetes, 1*(3), 76. https://doi.org/10.4239/wjd.v1.i3.76

Spritzler, F. (2019, April 24). *6 mistakes that slow down your metabolism.* Healthline. https://www.healthline.com/nutrition/6-mistakes-that-slow-metabolism#TOC_TITLE_HDR_2

Stockman, J. A. (2009). The spread of obesity in a large social network over 32 years. *Yearbook of Pediatrics, 2009,* 464–466. https://doi.org/10.1016/s0084-3954(08)79134-6

Stok, F. M., de Ridder, D. T. D., de Vet, E., & de Wit, J. B. F. (2013). Don't tell me what I should do, but what others do: The influence of descriptive and injunctive peer norms on fruit consumption in adolescents. *British Journal of Health Psychology, 19*(1), 52–64. https://doi.org/10.1111/bjhp.12030

Stress and eating. (2013). American Psychological Association. https://www.apa.org/news/press/releases/stress/2013/eating

Sweeney, E. (2021). What do doctors mean when they say "drink plenty of fluids"?. *Washington Post.* https://www.washingtonpost.com/lifestyle/2021/11/05/what-do-doctors-mean-when-they-say-drink-plenty-fluids/

10 surprising factors that affect your taste perception. (n.d.). Abbott. https://www.nutritionnews.abbott/news-research/expert-views/10-surprising-things-that-affect-your-taste/

The state of food security and nutrition in the world 2022. (2022). Food and Agriculture Organization of the United Nations. https://www.fao.

org/3/cc0639en/online/sofi-2022/cost-affordability-healthy-diet.html

Top tips for portion control. (2018, September 3). British Heart Foundation; British Heart Foundation. https://www.bhf.org.uk/informationsupport/heart-matters-magazine/nutrition/weight/perfect-portions/top-tips-for-portion-control

Trenkwalder, C., Hening, W. A., Montagna, P., Oertel, W. H., Allen, R. P., Walters, A. S., Costa, J., Stiasny-Kolster, K., & Sampaio, C. (2008). Treatment of restless legs syndrome: An evidence-based review and implications for clinical practice. *Movement Disorders, 23*(16), 2267–2302. https://doi.org/10.1002/mds.22254

van der Put, A., & Ellwardt, L. (2022). Employees' healthy eating and physical activity: the role of colleague encouragement and behaviour. *BMC Public Health, 22*(1). https://doi.org/10.1186/s12889-022-14394-0

Vartanian, L. R., Sokol, N., Herman, C. P., & Polivy, J. (2013). Social models provide a norm of appropriate food intake for young women. *PLoS ONE, 8*(11), e79268. https://doi.org/10.1371/journal.pone.0079268

Venter, C., Pereira, B., Grundy, J., Clayton, C. B., Arshad, S. H., & Dean, T. (2006). Prevalence of sensitization reported and objectively assessed food hypersensitivity amongst six-year-old children: A population-based study. *Pediatric Allergy and Immunology, 17*(5), 356–363. https://doi.org/10.1111/j.1399-3038.2006.00428.x

Vighi, G., Marcucci, F., Sensi, L., Di Cara, G., & Frati, F. (2008). Allergy and the gastrointestinal system. *Clinical & Experimental Immunology, 153*, 3–6. https://doi.org/10.1111/j.1365-2249.2008.03713.x

Vitamin and mineral supplements - what to know. (n.d.). Better Health Channel. https://www.betterhealth.vic.gov.au/health/healthyliving/vitamin-and-minerals

Vitamin C megadosage. (2023, January 29). Wikipedia. https://en.wikipedia.org/wiki/Vitamin_C_megadosage

Walsh, O. (2022). *Food deserts: What are they and what causes them.* The Human League. https://www.google.com/url?q=https://thehumaneleague.org/article/food-desert&sa=D&source=docs&ust=

1675358234562199&usg=AOvVaw0ElrFU-Bk64MlZUTsWDLTS

Water: how much should you drink every day? (2020, October 14). Mayo Clinic. https://www.mayoclinic.org/healthy-lifestyle/nutrition-and-healthy-eating/in-depth/water/art-20044256

Weight loss services in the US: market size 2003–2028. (2022). IBISWorld - Industry Market Research, Reports, and Statistics. https://www.ibisworld.com/industry-statistics/market-size/weight-loss-services-united-states/

Weight loss: choosing a diet that's right for you. (2018). Mayo Clinic. https://www.mayoclinic.org/healthy-lifestyle/weight-loss/in-depth/weight-loss/art-20048466

Weight loss: gain control of emotional eating. (2022). Mayo Clinic. https://www.mayoclinic.org/healthy-lifestyle/weight-loss/in-depth/weight-loss/art-20047342

What are proteins and what do they do? (2021, March 26). MedlinePlus. https://medlineplus.gov/genetics/understanding/howgeneswork/protein/

What is your attitude and relationship with food? (2021, July 20). Connectable Life Blog. https://www.connectablelife.com/blog/what-is-your-attitude-and-relationship-with-food/

Wilson, K. (2022). *Food aversion: A psychologist reveals why you hate some foods, but could learn to love them.* BBC Science Focus Magazine. https://www.sciencefocus.com/news/food-aversions/

Yt, L., Yh, C., Ms, L., & Ml, W. (2009). *Health and nutrition economics: diet costs are associated with diet quality.* Asia Pacific Journal of Clinical Nutrition. https://pubmed.ncbi.nlm.nih.gov/19965354/

Yu, H. (2017). *The psychology of restaurant interior design, part 2: scent.* Www.fohlio.com. https://www.fohlio.com/blog/the-psychology-of-restaurant-interior-design-part-2-scent

Zellner, D. A., Loss, C. R., Zearfoss, J., & Remolina, S. (2014). It tastes as good as it looks! The effect of food presentation on liking for the flavor of food ☆. *Appetite, 77,* 31–35. https://doi.org/10.1016/j.appet.2014.02.009

Zimmerle, D. (2022). *Are your friends influencing your food choices?*

Sharecare. https://www.sharecare.com/mens-health/peer-pres sure-and-eating-habits

Zopf, Y., Baenkler, H.-W., Silbermann, A., Hahn, E. G., & Raithel, M. (2009). The differential diagnosis of food intolerance. *Deutsches Aerzteblatt Online.* https://doi.org/10.3238/arztebl.2009.0359

IMAGE REFERENCES

Alisha Mishra. (2018). *Clear glass bottle filled with broccoli shake.* Pexels. https://www.pexels.com/photo/clear-glass-bottle-filled-with-broc coli-shake-1346347/

Andres Ayrton. (2021). *Asian athlete drinking water standing with bottle sports supplements.* Pexels. https://www.pexels.com/photo/asian-athlete-drinking-water-standing-with-bottle-sports-supplements-6551145/

Antony Trivet. (2022). *Plates with main courses on a table.* Pexels. https://www.pexels.com/photo/plates-with-main-courses-on-a-table-12842926/

Diva Plavalaguna. (2020). *Multiracial group of people by the table.* Pexels. https://www.pexels.com/photo/multiracial-group-of-people-by-the-table-6150432/

Geraud pfeiffer. (2021). *Plates with various raw meat with spices on table.* Pexels. https://www.pexels.com/photo/plates-with-various-raw-meat-with-spices-on-table-6607314/

Gustavo Fring. (2020). *Young businesswoman working remotely in cafe during lunch time.* Pexels. https://www.pexels.com/photo/young-businesswoman-working-remotely-in-cafe-during-lunch-time-3874618/

Jane Doan. (2018). *Assorted sliced fruits in white ceramic bowl.* Pexels. https://www.pexels.com/photo/assorted-sliced-fruits-in-white-ceramic-bowl-1092730/

JJ Jordan, (2022). *Paleo diet.* Pexels. https://www.pexels.com/photo/paleo-diet-10742586/

KoolShooters. (2021). *Girl eating a doughnut*. Pexels. https://www.pexels.com/photo/girl-eating-a-doughnut-7329720/

Lara Jameson. (2021). *Women setting up a table for traditional celebration*. Pexels. https://www.pexels.com/photo/women-setting-up-a-table-for-traditional-celebration-8887082/

Michaela. (2017). *Flat lay photography of unfold book beside macbook*. Pexels. https://www.pexels.com/photo/flat-lay-photography-of-unfold-book-beside-macbook-295826/

Moe Magners. (2021). *Papers with message hanging on the wall*. Pexels. https://www.pexels.com/photo/papers-with-message-hanging-on-the-wall-6669475/

RODNAE Productions. (2021). *Close-up shot of a spring roll*. Pexels. https://www.pexels.com/photo/close-up-shot-of-a-spring-roll-6646372/

Pixabay. (2017). Blue tape measuring on clear glass square weighing scale. Pexels. https://www.pexels.com/photo/blue-tape-measuring-on-clear-glass-square-weighing-scale-53404/

Pixabay. (2017). *Bowl being poured with yellow liquid*. Pexels. https://www.pexels.com/photo/bowl-being-poured-with-yellow-liquid-33783/

ROMBO. (2020). *Measuring guitar pick*. Pexels. https://www.pexels.com/photo/measuring-guitar-pick-3988555/

Shopify Partners. (n.d.). *A nurse makes some adjustments to a weight apparatus*. Burst. https://burst.shopify.com/photos/nurse-operating-weight-apparatus?q=weight

Shopify Partners. (n.d.). [Teal ribbon]. Burst. https://burst.shopify.com/photos/teal-ribbon-center?q=teal+ribbon

Vanessa Loring. (2020). *A person holding a plastic container with bread and biscuits*. Pexels. https://www.pexels.com/photo/a-person-holding-a-plastic-container-with-bread-and-biscuits-5971867/

Vegan Liftz. (2019). *Blue ceramic plate with meal plan blocks*. Pexels. https://www.pexels.com/photo/blue-ceramic-plate-with-meal-plan-blocks-2377165/

www.ingramcontent.com/pod-product-compliance
Lightning Source LLC
Chambersburg PA
CBHW030410130626
46549CB00004B/1703